Reviews

"I sincerely hope she will continue her role as an educator, relating her experiences not only to those individuals that are recent victims of stroke, but also to health care professionals and students who seek to understand the patient's perspective."

–Mario deFigueiredo, Ph.D.

Fellow, Institute of Food Technologists

"In my experience, I found it interesting to see how a strong independent professional woman dealt with disability and struggled to maintain her independence. Through her hard work, determination and the support of her husband and friends she made great improvements in her function. Professionally, I think all rehabilitation professionals could benefit from reading such an account."

–Anne Doroba, M.D.

Physiatrist

SWIMMING AGAINST THE TIDE: STRONG RECOVERY FROM STROKE

Nan Unklesbay, Ph.D.

Published by AKA:yoLa / AKA-Publishing
Columbia, Missouri
www.akayola.com

"Opportunity" by Walter Malone is reprinted from The Little Book of American Poets: 1787-1900. Ed. Jessie B. Rittenhouse. Cambridge: Riverside Press, 1915.

Cover and Interior design by Bryan Farevaag

Library of Congress
Unklesbay, Nan
Swimming Against The Tide: Strong Recovery from Stroke
1. Stroke 2. Heart surgery 3. Myxoma 4. Occupational therapy 5. Physical therapy 6. Speech therapy 7. Self help

ISBN-13: 978-0-9842288-7-4
ISBN-10: 0-9842288-7-X

AKA-Publishing
AKA:yoLa

SWIMMING AGAINST THE TIDE: STRONG RECOVERY FROM STROKE

Nan Unklesbay, Ph.D.

Contents

Acknowledgements

I appreciate the care I received at Boone Hospital Center, in Columbia, Missouri. They gave me knowledge to enhance the quality of my life.
I would also like to express my deep appreciation to the following:

Douglas E. Vogt, M.D., the Internal Medicine Physician who continues to take care of my medical needs.

David L. McLaren, M.D., the Neurologist who directed my activities within the Rehabilitation Unit and continues to take care of my neurological needs.

Richard J. Mellitt, M.D., the Cardiovascular Surgeon who removed my myxoma.

Tony J. Spaedy, M.D., the Cardiologist who continues to take care of my heart-related needs.

In memory of Leland V. Pfefer, M.D. who was my Family Physician when my myxoma was discovered.

To all of the Physical, Occupational, Speech and Rehabilitation Therapists at Boone Hospital Center. All were so patient with me. I give special thanks to Jeri Marine, M.S., my Speech Pathologist who taught me math skills. My nickname for her was "the professor," as she challenged me.

So many other people and professionals to thank!

Special thanks and appreciation go to my lifelong friends, Nordis Milne, an Occupational and Physical Therapist, and Barbara Mulhern, a Special Education teacher. Many thanks to Heather R. Huhman and Noreen Curry for technical assistance, and to Regiena Lopez, Janet Musick and Yvonne Skouby for editing.

My brother, who was my only passenger when I was terrified to drive in the dark, and for his great, continual support.

My cousin, Regiena and her husband, Ruben who frequently brought their children (Micaela, Gabrilla, Alexandra and Olivia) to the Rehabilitation Unit to visit me. Ruben shared pharmacy advice with me.

My current Physical Therapist, Rick Rother, P.T. CEAS.

Beverly Miles, D.C., my Chiropractor who gives me ongoing treatment, advice and guidance.
Paula Thomas, our Travel Agent at Great South-

ern Travel, Columbia, Missouri, who never gets us lost!

My former students who encouraged me from many parts of the world.

In memory of my friend, Richard E. Knox, M.D., who encouraged me during my recoveries from heart surgery and a stroke.

My extended family, for their special love, concern and care.

My friends and colleagues, for their motivation during my recoveries.

Rev. Jim Bryan, my former Pastor at Missouri United Methodist Church in Columbia, Missouri, whose sermons helped with my connection to God.

Finally, I thank my supportive husband, Kenneth, whose love and help with my daily life made it possible for me to write this book.

Opportunity

When I left my parents' home in North Vancouver, British Columbia, to take a position in St. John's, Newfoundland, Canada, my mother gave me a framed copy of this poem:

OPPORTUNITY

They do me wrong who say I come no more
When once I knock and fail to find you in;
For every day I stand outside your door
And bid you wake, and rise to fight and win.

Wail not for precious chances passed away!
Weep not for golden ages on the wane!
Each night I burn the records of the day--
At sunrise every soul is born again!

–Walter Malone (1866-1915)

I have frequently read this poem since I had a stroke. To me, this means I face new challenges every day. Somebody is watching me so I will do as well as I can. I will exert myself as much as I am able. If I do not try hard enough, all is forgiven, because the next day I will face the same challenges again. I hope you can benefit from these words as much as I have.

To My Readers

I wrote this book after I had an embolism, commonly known as a stroke, on the right side of my brain. My left side was affected, as well as my math and logic abilities. All strokes are different, but the one thing they have in common is that your attention span is affected. It frustrates me that I now think so slowly.

This book is intended for those of you who have had a stroke and are able to read, or are assisting a person who has had a stroke. Much of the information can also be used by those who have head injuries from an accident or who are suffering from traumatic brain injury (TBI). This book is a diligent account of my recovery process. If you have had a stroke and cannot concentrate for very long, I suggest, at first, you read small parts of this book at each sitting, concentrating on parts that interest you the most. I have sections throughout called "Your Enlightenment," which are essentially "take-aways" from each chapter.

I wrote *Swimming Against the Tide* because a couple of dear friends, one of whom is an occupational and physical therapist, suggested I do so because there aren't many books available written by people who have recovered from a stroke. This is because most stroke victims are not able to write a book. My friends thought it would help others who had suffered a stroke to be able to share another patient's experiences. Since I have written books before, I decided to accept this challenge.

As a college professor, my previous writing experiences had been academic ones in which I related results of research projects. For this book, I had to learn to write in first person and share my emotions, a very different form of writing than to which I had been accustomed. Many people write books with a second author who is a professional writer; I wrote this book alone. Writing to you has been therapeutic for me, as I had to document and reflect on everything that has happened.

My recovery is continually in progress. I had heard about people who had strokes, but had no knowledge of what it would be like to recover. I hope I have covered all issues that will be of concern to you. I have given specific details that can aid your recovery from a stroke.

I am aware that every stroke is different and requires different medications and therapies. Your sense of humor will be helpful to you, as mine has been to me. I hope you continue to have as positive an outlook on your future life as I have on mine. I wish you the best of luck in getting there. You will make it!

There were numerous reasons for choosing the title of this book, *Swimming Against the Tide:*

Strong Recovery from Stroke. Strokes and tides occur around the globe, so my hope is that this book can be used to educate students in health care professions and inspire patients facing recovery through placement in rehabilitation facilities, libraries, and availability in bookstores around the globe.

Before my stroke, I was a very strong swimmer, but I swam in two tides that were too strong for me. I was strong enough to swim out of them, but their terrifying memories will remain with me. First, I was swimming in a Norwegian fjiord with a friend. Our purpose was to observe houses near hers that I had never seen before. We swam against a very strong tide and finally made it, exhausted, back to her home. Second, just after my mother died, I was swimming in the Burrard Inlet near West Vancouver, British Columbia, Canada. As I was upset, I swam too far away from shore. A fellow swimmer realized I had gone too far, and she came to swim with me back to shore. I was sure glad to be back to Ambleside Beach in West

Vancouver.

My recovery from my stroke is a long one. I am still swimming against a tide, confident I will continue to improve. This effort is constant.

I was swimming when I had my stroke. Luckily, I was in a pool without any tides. I have been able to swim again for exercise since my stroke. Mentally, I have written most of this book for you as I do my laps. I hope my global readers do everything they can do to carry forward and have the level of persistence they need to thrust forward without having detours (not swimming against the tide). Partners and spouses can use the phrase "swimming against the tide" to encourage those recovering from strokes to try to make good progress to undo the effects of a stroke, as much as mentally and physically possible.

How I Got Here

Since this book is a description of my personal experiences and feelings during a portion of my life, I think it would be helpful to give you a brief history of how I got to this point.

I was born in North Vancouver, British Columbia, Canada, on March 28, 1944. I graduated from high school in 1962. My guidance counselor explained that I had poor scores on my university entrance examinations and should not consider attending a university, especially for dietetics, which required extensive science courses. My Norwegian father agreed with him. His philosophy was I should soon get married and have a husband to support me. I defied them both and enrolled at the University of British Columbia (UBC) in 1962. I struggled, as I have since seen many students do. I graduated with my Bachelor of Science degree in Dietetics in 1966.

In 1967, I moved to Toronto for a one year dietetic internship at Toronto Western Hospital. After completing the internship, I accepted a position at St. John's in Newfoundland, Canada, with the Department of Health as a dietary consultant. By that time, I had a wonderful mentor, my supervisor, who was guiding my career. My office was at the eastern end of the Trans Canada Highway and the opposite end of the country; I was as far away from home as I could get and still be in Canada. My job was to visit all the cottage hospitals throughout Newfoundland and Labrador to give them advice about dietetics. In one hospital in Labrador, I was working with the Inuit. They did not have an understanding of sanitation, but through my teachings, they understood and accepted the concepts well. I really enjoyed my position and, after one year, I had saved enough money so that I could travel to Europe and visit my relatives in Norway, Scotland, and England.

After three years, my mentor said she thought I had done all I could do in Newfoundland at the time, and she urged me to consider getting my Master of Science degree. I enrolled at the University of Wisconsin in Madison in the Department of Food Science. After some intense studying, I received my M.S. degree in Food Science in 1971 and my Ph.D. degree in Food Science in 1973. When I came home to North Vancouver with my Ph.D., my father could not have been more pleased. Apparently, I had changed his mind about the role of women!

I accepted a position as Assistant Professor at the University of Missouri in Columbia, Missouri (UMC) in the Department of Food Science. I met my future husband, Ken, who was an Assistant Professor in Electrical Engineering, also at UMC. When people ask me why I remained here after coming from beautiful Vancouver, I say "love."

My academic life was fun. I worked on exciting research projects. Sometimes Ken and I combined our efforts and researched food-engineering problems. I had my first experience as an author in 1982 when Ken and I wrote a book entitled, *Energy Management in Foodservice.* My second experience came in 1992 when I wrote a book entitled *World Food and You*. I taught a course by that name for a number of years. I wanted students to understand the dynamic world food situation.

The highlight of my career occurred when I was

featured in the January 3-10, 2000 issue of *U. S. News and World Report* as one of eighteen "Innovators of the Millennium" for my public health research. At that time, I was engaged in research on food irradiation with my graduate students.

Everything was in my future. I enjoyed my academic position at a good university. I had a wonderful husband I shared with our two Russian Blue cats. I had a caring extended family and wonderful friends and colleagues.

I hope my research and teaching efforts have a positive influence on the future. I always enjoy contact with my previous students. Sometimes they tell me that things I said to them have made a significant difference in their lives.

A routine physical in February 2000 found a myxoma in the left atrium of my heart. A myxoma is a tumor that is usually benign but can grow to fill the heart cavity. In order to prevent a fatal stoke, it was removed by open-heart surgery at Boone Hospital Center on February 26, 2000. The tumor was found to be benign. As I recovered, I slowly got stronger and returned to my teaching and research responsibilities in August 2000.

On December 31, 2002, my husband and I took advantage of an early retirement plan. My plans were to participate in an international committee for the Institute of Food Technologists (IFT).

On February 26, 2003, I had a stroke while I was swimming alone. After my stroke, which was on the right side of my brain, physicians found I had a high blood-clotting factor. The left side of my body was affected. Fortunately, I did not have any paralysis. My speech was not affected. My main disability was I could no longer work with numbers and had trouble with logical thinking. I had spent my life doing research as a professor, usually using statistics, and had written more than 100 scientific papers, but I lost this ability. Luckily, I had retired!

I was fortunate to spend one month in the inpatient rehabilitation ward at Boone Hospital Center in Columbia, Missouri, followed by outpatient therapy and learning how to adjust at home.

Although I am still recovering, nobody can tell I have had a stroke unless they ask me a question involving numbers or logical sequences. The following chapters focus on my life after suffering a stroke when I was 59 years old.

1

One: Getting Healthy And Fit

I chose the title of this chapter to imply I was not always fit. To use a Canadian phrase, I finally "smartened up" and did what I could to become healthy.

When I graduated with my bachelor's degree, I was 22 years old. I knew what to eat, and I knew I should exercise. Knowing something and doing something do not always coincide. When I was 35 years old, I became ill with shingles and soon realized I had to get strong and fit. I was ashamed of that 13-year delay. All I can say is that life's commitments overwhelmed me, and I ignored the basic knowledge gained from the education I was proud to have the opportunity to initiate and acquire.

There is no question that a proper diet and exercise are important to having good health. In the developed world we live in, we are bombarded with information on diet and exercise, some sound and some not. Over the years, people have become more aware of the value of good nutrition and exercise in maintaining their health and are more conscientious about their behavior. On the other hand, the level of obesity in our society has continued to increase. Since this is a complex issue and there are many other sources of information on these subjects, I am not going to elaborate other than to give you some of my personal observations and experiences from having worked as a food scientist and dietitian for many years.

As the food industry strives to formulate and market more new foods, the processes involved in their production have become more technically complex. For example, to keep costs down, there has been more emphasis on the use of by-products. Also, there has been more technology used on farms to produce higher yields at lower cost. More foods from foreign sources have been imported. Foods are being formulated to respond to the changing dietary habits of consumers. The demand for foods that are quick and easy to prepare, fat-free, low in carbohydrates, and high in fiber have made grocery shopping a complex activity. Also, we eat in a larger variety of locations than in the past, requiring foods that can be served in these settings.

These demands cause new, complex problems to occur. We now are not only affected by the foods we eat but by the feeds our food ate. The use of aquaculture has produced farm-raised fish, and some contain pesticide residues obtained from their food. The modern diets for cattle have produced Bovine Spongiform Encephalopathy (BSE), commonly referred to as Mad Cow Disease. I have followed these developments over the years and have been amazed at the complexity of the problems that have been discovered. I am sure there are more to come.

This makes knowing what you should eat a very frustrating situation. When we are continually given new and often conflicting information about nutrition, how can we know that we are eating the right foods? This is a problem for which I do not have a complete answer. With my academic background, you are probably asking why I cannot give you a good answer. All that I can say is that good, sound research is continuing, and more answers will be available in the future. Today, we should believe advice that nutritionists and food scientists share with us.

Who are Food Scientists?

As I was formerly a food scientist, I wish to define our activities to you.

The profession of food science is a rather obscure profession, as most people are not aware of the benefits we offer to our fast-moving society. Students take courses in microbiology, biology, chemistry, nutrition, genetic engineering, physics, and engineering. Food scientists are mostly employed in food processing plants where they prepare quality food with acceptable levels of sanitation for extended shelf times. Food Scientists are responsible for analyzing the nutrients labeled "Nutrition Facts" on food packaging and containers.

As some nutrients degrade with time, food scientists design food processes to ensure the nutrients are in your foods when you consume them. During the last thirty years, I taught students who now work in food processing plants across the U.S., Canada, and Mexico. I have no doubt you have bought products in which some of my students were involved.

Some food scientists measure microbial quality, while others measure food quality, which includes sensory aspects and nutrients. Every food product has to meet our food laws, so others are responsible for enforcing national and international food laws. We want your foods to be safe, good tasting, and to contain desired nutrients to benefit your nutritional health.

I am sure by now you realize how excited I was about my profession. Educating undergraduate and graduate students was a rewarding experience. Many of my former Ph.D. students are now professors in other food science departments.

Every individual's health profile is determined by genetics and behavioral factors. As you know, the leading adult causes of death are cancer, heart disease, stroke, injuries, and chronic lung disease. Changing unhealthy habits to healthy ones can improve the quality of life for adults and lessen the chance of disability. For example, incorporating exercise and a balanced low-fat diet into one's lifestyle contributes to weight loss and controls risk factors for heart disease. Having a high fat intake, being overweight, and not getting enough exercise increase your health risk. With all of life's glorious opportunities, why settle for a boring, sedentary life?

Nutrition alone is not enough to prevent many diseases, but it certainly helps. Plan to exercise regularly if you are motivated to maintain good health as you age. Even a ten-minute walk each day is better than not walking at all. With persistence, great improvement can be achieved. Exercise causes muscle improvement and more blood flow to your brain. A major benefit of regular exercise is, as energy output increases, you can eat more food and obtain more nutrients. As calorie needs decrease with age, the need for certain nutrients such as calcium, Vitamin D, Vitamin C, Vitamin B_{12}, and Vitamin B_6 actually increase. I take Centrum Silver™ and Natural Factors™ with calcium, magnesium, potassium, manganese. I also take Carlson™ Cod Liver Oil and Carlson™ Vitamin D drops daily in addition to my balanced diet. It is also important to remember to consume six to eight glasses of water per day, especially for older adults.

Exercising to Get Fit

When I was young, people did not exercise for the sake of getting exercise. Exercise was a by-product of some other activity. I grew up on the coast of the Pacific Ocean and swam at an early age, but only for fun, not for exercise. When I was in college, I was too busy studying and having a good time. I did not have time for exercise.

When I got married, my father was concerned that I was not exercising and gave me a rowing machine for a wedding present. I ignored his advice and did not use it. A few years after I started working at the University of Missouri, stress from my career caused me to get shingles. At that time, medicines now used to treat the disease were not available, and my recovery was long and painful. As I recovered, I was too weak to walk the block around our home. I learned to relax more and used self-hypnosis to control my stress level, but realized I had to get more physically fit.

My physician at the time was a marathon runner, and he suggested I jog on a regular basis. I purchased new shoes and a jogging outfit and went to the university gym where I met other women with the same condition as mine. Eventually, we all ran a 7K marathon, and I finished last. I was not accustomed to finishing last, so I persisted and realized getting up early each morning to jog was actually enjoyable. I started to feel much better as my strength improved. As a bonus, I made good new friends in the process. Since I loved to swim and it was easier on my joints, I joined a country club with a swimming pool and swam every day after work during the summers. At that time of day, the children had all gone home and only a few dedicated swimmers were there. In the winters, I went to a gym that had a pool and continued to swim every day. During that time, my health and fitness improved dramatically.

Physically Building Our Home

In 1987, Ken and I bought 22 acres in the country and decided to build a house. We had never discussed what type of house we wanted. We received an issue of *Homes* and we both became excited about a house in Arkansas. The architect worked for Fay Jones, who was a student of Frank

Lloyd Wright. I loved the Frank Lloyd Wright homes I had seen near Madison, Wisconsin, and both Ken and I enjoyed the Guggenheim Museum in New York City.

We drove to Arkansas to meet John Womack, the architect featured in the magazine. He showed us several of his houses in the area, and we became enthused. We returned home and read several books about designing homes. We spent two weeks at the dining room table laying out our plans. I did not like John's kitchens, so I laid out a floor plan for ours.

Several months later, John came to Columbia. It was wonderful to see an architect walking our land and "designing in his head." John read our plans and designed our home.

When we returned to Arkansas to see the floor plans, we found that we could not afford the home we planned and had to make compromises. For example, we had planned a lookout as the top floor, which we did not need. So, Ken sent John a new set of blueprints with our latest wishes.

John frequently said that Ken is the only owner who had ever sent him any blueprints. After three years, we had 36 pages of blueprints of a home we liked and could afford.

This book is about my recovery from a stroke, not about building a house. However, a large portion of my overall fitness today can be attributed to work I put into building our home. Perhaps, if it were not for these efforts, I would not have recovered from my stroke as well as I have. When we started out, both Ken and I did not know we would have to work so hard. We had a complex plan and could not find contractors to work at a reasonable price and complete all the details we demanded. Luckily, both Ken and I were fit and able.

Many people say, "We built our home." However, Ken and I always say we "physically built our home."

After purchasing our land, we spent considerable time clearing scrub and old fences, as it had been untended farm land.

After the clearing was done, we bought trees from the Conservation Department and planted and maintained them. Our summers were hot, so we spent considerable time watering them and installing wires on stakes to prevent deer from eating them.

We moved hay bales and began the mowing process. I refused to learn how to drive a tractor, as the bouncing terrified me. I spent many times in sheer terror, just screaming as I tried. So, Ken totally took over the mowing job.

During weekends and summers from 1990 to 1997, Ken and I did much of the construction work ourselves on our 7,000-square foot home, which included concrete patios that made it easy to entertain. Because of my prior exercise regime, I was able to do this kind of work. My nail-hammering ability never excelled, so I was instructed never to drive nails that would show when our home was finished. I spent hours and hours on scaffolding, keeping my balance. My graduate students would come to "our site" at night for help with their laboratory problems. I became known as "the burro."

I carried lumber from our truck and trailer to our site. I helped place the large overhead beams. Fortunately, Ken used winches to help with the process. I helped lift walls that were framed on the floor and heaved into place. By the time we were ready to place to our bedroom wall, I remember heaving and saying, "Why am I doing this?"

We had a brick mason lay all the brick. However, he did not want to make mortar to fill the concrete blocks, so that became my responsibility. The concrete blocks around our home extended from 2 to 12 feet deep. In September 1993, I started mixing sand, cement, and gravel in a concrete mixer. I can vividly remember reading "made in Winnipeg" as the mixer turned. I usually worked like a professor, taking extreme care with chemical and biological formulas. I had to learn to judge the right amount of ingredients, largely based on the weather and how much rain we had. We were experiencing the "100 year flood" of the Missouri River, and our property was constantly muddy! In the beginning, I struggled to carry one bucket of mortar to its correct place, anywhere from 2 to 20 feet. By May, I could easily carry two buckets. I dug a lot of mud. I remember one morning scraping mud from concrete blocks, changing clothes, and then going to work. My undergraduate students and colleagues had no idea how I started my morning.

My level of fitness meant I was physically strong, had good balance, and had great stamina. Still, I occasionally fell in thick mud, which infuriated me. I worked as a burro and could find anything Ken directed me to locate.

There was not one day we decided we could not work, except during our cold winters, when Ken read our blueprints and made plans for the spring. On one hot, humid day, we had to quit working at 2 p.m. We went home and slept and were back working by 7 p.m. For seven years, I had no trouble sleeping.

With this total commitment, Ken and I agreed we would not travel. On two occasions, I realized I needed a break. I traveled with one of my girlfriends twice for a week to recuperate and have a good time. I lied about where I was going. I came back much refreshed and ready to go again. Ken never found out about my travels and will not until he reads this book. At the time, I guess I just felt desperate for a "normal life."

I was not always patient during this building process. Ken is a perfectionist. On one occasion, I remember we had to decide on the angle of a board. I said, "Make it 45 degrees." Ken used geometry and calculated that it should be 44.6 degrees. As our saw would not cut at 44.6 degrees, he sawed it at 45 degrees. I exceeded my frustration level many times, but was able to continue because I had set a goal. A basic part of my character is that I am persistent in achieving my goals.

As we worked with our architect, I talked Ken into building our lap pool. At the time, we had no idea my health problems would make this such a good idea. When we finished, Ken had to learn pool management and maintenance, but it cut down on the time I wasted coming and going to a pool because we now had our own ten feet from our bedroom. I swam half a mile each day and was fit and in good health. I would not recommend anyone follow this strenuous exercise plan, but it worked for me.

Your Enlightenment

Despite being fit, I had heart surgery and later a stroke. After each of these events, I worried I had done something wrong to cause my condition or that I could have done something to prevent it. I have had a lot of anguish about these feelings but have come to learn that even very fit and healthy people can have severe medical problems through no fault of their own. In my case, the myxoma removed from my heart was a very rare condition and the cause is unknown. I did not cause it, and I could not have prevented it. After my stroke, I found I have a higher clotting factor than normal. Again, it was not my fault, and I could not have prevented it. Sometimes events just happen, as they did to me. I will continue to enjoy a long life.

After my heart surgery, I exercised as much as I could. I do not have high blood pressure, and my cholesterol values are good. Also, results from a stress test two years after my heart surgery showed excellent values. I believe my level of fitness made shortened my recovery time. I have continued to exercise since my stroke and now have nearly no physical disability.

When I go to physicians today, they admire my physical strength, which makes me feel good. I am not saying you have to physically build a house to get strong, but you should find a form of exercise you can do consistently.

When one has heart surgery or a stroke, one has a current physical state. If you are strong and have a good level of health and fitness, you will recover much more fully and faster. Once an event like this occurs, you cannot go back in time and change things. There is no healing value in anguishing over what you should have done. Deal with the future. If you need to change your diet or level of fitness, start to do so immediately. Please continue with the advice your physicians give you. I am sure they have advised you to stay healthy and fit. There are numerous articles and references with advice you can ask about. Please do not start a new diet or exercise program without your health professional's advice.

2

Two: Recovering from Open-Heart Surgery

In February 2000, my family physician ordered a CT (computed tomography) scan of my pancreas because I had hypoglycemia, (episodes of low blood sugar.) While reviewing the CT results, the radiologist found my pancreas was fine, but I had an abnormal growth inside my heart. It was a myxoma in the left atrium of my heart, which is a very rare type of tumor. It had to be removed because it could continue to grow and eventually obstruct the flow of blood throughout my heart. You cannot imagine the terror I had when I got a phone call from my physician telling me what had been found. He told me a heart surgeon had just moved to town to take care of difficult heart problems, such as mine. I learned a piece of a myxoma, or blood clots that form on the surface of the myxoma, may cut off circulation to other organs and cause blocked blood vessels. Symptoms depend on which vessel is blocked. If a vessel to the brain is involved, a fatal stroke can occur. The surgeon had seen only a few myxomas, as they are so rare. I had to trust his competence.

I was given the pre-operation tests, which found nothing else wrong with my heart. I remember my cardiologist saying, "We don't want to remove the myxoma and later find you need a by-pass operation. We want the whole job done in one operation." After the tests were done, he said, "You have the arteries of an 18-year-old."

The pre-op visit that surprised me most was with the anesthesiologist. I thought they just administered anesthesia and did not have contact with patients. He described different kinds of medication he would be using, but then told me he did not know whether he was scheduled for my surgery. Later, when I was wheeled into the operating room, he was there. It was a relief to know someone I had met and liked was going to be taking care of me.

Prior to my surgery, I was scheduled to have my annual evaluation with my University Department Chairperson. She expected to review my past year's work, but I interrupted her to tell her my news. She said, "You look terrible, how can I help?" I said, "You have a problem. Someone has to teach my classes while I am gone." That was my last day at work for seven months. I had a week to wait with the dread of surgery hanging over my head. I had to have a lawyer write my power of attorney. I had to give blood in case it was needed during the operation. I had an interview at the hospital, which can best be described as a psychological examination. At last, they decided I was ready for surgery.

My operation was scheduled for early in the morning on February 26, 2000, just one week after the myxoma had been identified. The night before the heart surgery, I had a long swim, talked to family and friends, and got a good night's sleep. I had done my research, I knew the surgery was necessary, and had confidence in my surgeon. When the anesthetic was beginning to take effect, I apparently said, "Let's get this over with." A nurse told Ken having a positive attitude would really help me.

Soon, I realized I was still alive and very groggy in the Intensive Care Unit (ICU). Ken said I looked like I was dead. A nurse assured me I would be fine, and she would stay with me. My operation had taken four hours. It was a short time for me but a long time for my husband and two friends, who were waiting at the hospital.

While I was in the ICU, I was connected to tubes and wires. I had a tube in my throat, so I could not talk. I became very frustrated trying to communicate with gestures when I could hardly move. I had several visitors, including the Dean of my College. He gave me a very warm greeting. Whenever I have seen him since, I remember that visit because it meant so much to me. After I had a stroke, his wife also came for a cheery visit. She encouraged me not to be too negative. They really left an impression on me. When I got out of the ICU, I was put in a hospital room for two days to recover. The visitors I had were really appreciated. From this experience, I have learned to be a frequent hospital visitor, since I now know how much it means to a patient.

Regaining My Strength

My surgeon visited me numerous times while I was in my hospital room and seemed pleased with my progress. During one visit, he distracted me and pulled the drain tube out of my chest all in one yank. I hope I never feel such pain again. I guess if he had told me he was going to do that, it would have been worse. I still have a little round scar on my chest where the tube had been. The staff made me walk right away with a support person. After two days, I was discharged. This seemed like a very short time, considering the severity of my condition.

As Ken drove me home, he looked petrified that he would have to take care of me in that condition along with every thing else he had to do. A nurse called for the next several days. She was particularly interested in my breathing. I had to use a lung capacity meter to make sure my lungs were starting to recover. This device was a cylinder with a yellow ball inside that measured the amount of air taken in when I inhaled through the tube.

I was on medication for intense pain, and was given a heart-shaped pillow that I held tightly to my chest when I coughed. It lessened the pain, but unfortunately I developed bronchitis, which increased the amount of coughing. Since then, several friends whose spouses had open-heart surgery have been very cautious about visitors. Bronchitis after surgery was especially uncomfortable since breathing was terribly painful.

I was very weak and laid in bed most of the time. I had a bell to ring when I needed anything, and I am sure I abused this service. Ken walked me around the house. Due to our home being built on one level, I did not have any stairs to climb. Our two offices are in a loft, and I had no need to climb the stairs to visit my office. I was given a schedule for walking that required me to walk farther each day.

Finding a comfortable sitting position in bed was hard. Our two cats, Sorrento and Sointula, spent their days lying on the bed with me, and I enjoyed their company. They never had it so good. Ken cooked our meals and took care of the house, only leaving me alone when he had to go to the University.

As I had been physically fit, no physical therapy was recommended. I spent my days in bed reading, taking phone calls, stroking cats, watching television, and enjoying visits from friends. I was bored, and the pain was intense, but I knew I had to take the medication and deal with it.

I hated being inside all of the time. Of course, I felt sorry for myself. I thought of others who were house bound, and empathized with them. I just had to believe I would eventually get stronger. The people around me helped improve my state of mind. I had visits from many friends who brought food and news from the outside world. Our house is still full of houseplants that were given to me at the time. I have kept most of them alive.

Enjoying Scenery

After about a month, I felt strong enough to go outdoors. My physician was pleased with my healing progress and my heart sounded good. I was able to drive again but did not feel like driving very far.

While I had been lying in bed, I watched two blue herons on our pond. I decided to go see them close up. I slowly walked to the pond, which was 600 feet from our house. The first things I saw were two baby blue herons, which had probably hatched while I was lying in bed. They were frightened of me and splashed around in our pond. I presume they later grew up and flew away.

We had built a three-quarter mile grass jogging

trail around our property. When the grass started to turn green, my first effort was to walk on this trail. Some days I made 600 feet and some days I made 1200 feet, but I was always careful to be sure I could make it back to the house when I got too tired. I did not need constant attention, but a dear friend called me at 2 o'clock every afternoon to see if I was okay. I looked forward to her calls. As spring came, the grass turned green, the leaves budded on trees, the wildflowers started to grow, and I scared wildlife. Wild turkeys flew away, and white-tailed deer ran from me. The robins returned, and the turtles became active. The rabbits and squirrels played around me. The times I spent walking and observing the trail reminded me of an assignment I had done in British Columbia as a Girl Guide when I had to observe all the activities of nature in several acres of woods for one year.

It was a happy day when I was able to walk around the complete trail. This occurred in August when a cousin from Calgary walked with me. I wore a heart rate monitor so I could make sure my heart rate did not get too high.

Nature is especially important to me, and it certainly was on those days. I took pictures around the trail, which I displayed on my bulletin board when I returned to the University. The sign on my bulletin board said, "Come and Get Healthy With Me."

Ken and I always combine Canada Day (July 1,) with Independence Day and celebrate with a large party. My good friend from Wisconsin asked if she could help. She makes the most gorgeous cakes, so I asked her to bring one. A friend from the University who is a meat scientist prepared some wonderful barbequed pork, and his dear wife cleaned up the mess. Ken assumed his traditional job of making sure the fireworks did not set the house on fire. I didn't have to do anything but have a good time and enjoy my friends.

In the middle of the summer, Ken had a serious talk with me because I was being selfish, thinking my condition was the most important thing. I was not being a team player. He knew I was not as strong as I had been, but I was not as feeble as I was acting. I had gotten too used to being waited on all the time. The message really stung. I was not aware I was acting so dependent. His message hit home, and I started to do more for myself and not be such a burden.

Swimming After Heart Surgery

As swimming is a major part of my fitness regime, I bought a bathing suit that would hide the large scar on my chest. I wanted to swim as soon as possible. Our pool is seventy-five feet long, five feet deep, and ten feet wide. It is covered with a dome from the first of October to the end of May so I can swim year-round. The water is heated and kept at 80° F.

I was accustomed to swimming in cold water. I learned to swim in Vancouver, and we swam when the ocean temperature finally reached 68° F. I remember the radio announcer used to say, "It is time to swim."

I have swum across the fjords near Bergen, Norway, and off the northernmost tip of Newfoundland. Now, I wanted the pool at 80° F.

After my surgery, I was afraid to get into the pool because I was not sure I could climb up the steps to get out. I expressed my concern to my chiropractor, and she treated me with magnet therapy. I soon found I was strong enough. A friend came to swim with me every day for seven weeks just to be sure I did not drown. My chest really hurt when I swam, so I began swimming on alternate days to ease the pain. Some of my friends thought it was ridiculous to endure such pain, but swimming had always been such a major part of my life that I wanted to continue with it. As the saying goes, "No pain, no gain."

So, with time, I was able to swim routinely again. My swimming strokes were the same as ever, but I did not have sufficient energy to swim the half-mile per day I had previously done. Occasionally, I overdid it, and my chest pain returned. It reminded me I was not fully back to normal.

Returning to Work

I returned on a hot, humid day in August 2000 to teach my class, World Food and You, to 130 undergraduate students. On the first day, I felt so weak I did not know if I would make it indoors to the podium. I did not want any of my students to know I was recovering from surgery. I still had a condition common in patients who have had heart surgery—saying completely the wrong word without knowing I said it. Stress, such as teaching to so many students, increases this effect. I hoped I would conduct myself appropriately.

Information in the class dealt with the dynamic world food situation. My goal was to competently teach students, giving them current information. That semester, the war started in Afghanistan, so their assignment was to become familiar with how food aid was flown in to the people. *Foreign Affairs* had always been part of my reading material, and I had been reading it as I recovered from open-heart surgery.

In such a large class, there is a wide variety of

students. Some students are more serious than others, and it is sometimes a challenge to keep order. Students usually focus on what is going on in their lives and are not aware professors have situations of their own.

Two girls sat in the first row beside each other, directly in front of me. They were not always attentive and passed notes to each other. After watching this for a while, I sent them both e-mails telling them I had recently had heart surgery and hoped I was not confusing them when I said the wrong words. One of them sent me a card that said, "We enjoy your class because you give us current ideas, and we are amazed that you can teach such a large class with so much vigor after your heart surgery." They continued to sit in the same seats, but gave me their constant attention. At first, I had tried to go on as if nothing had happened, but I found people were helpful and understanding once they knew my situation.

One of my graduate students had been waiting for my return. So we restarted our research project, which had been put on hold. The project was funded before I had surgery, so luckily I did not have to seek additional research funds. We finished the food quality project, and my student was able to graduate in May 2002. The results of our research project were published the next fall, and he was offered a good job with the Food and Drug Administration (FDA).

My return to the University was successful. I received good teaching evaluations from students and a special graduate student received his M.S. degree and accepted a good job. By achieving the personal goals I had set for myself, I felt I had successfully recovered from open-heart surgery!

A Special Friend

A good Norwegian friend came to stay with us for two months. Although she had been through some troubling times of her own, she had the lovely Scandinavian spirit that can get you through each day. She kept me motivated to do as much as I could. By that time, I was teaching and performing research. She cooked several of our meals and suggested we party all the time. We had a warm fall, so she enjoyed being able to get a tan, until the weather got too cold. We had a busy two months. I had little time to think about the fact that I was recovering. Looking back on those two months, I really appreciated the help she gave me. Her visit came at the right time.

Traveling Again

Ken and I traveled to Norway, the Shetland Islands, Scotland, and the remote Faeroe Islands, north of Scotland, in July 2002. When I think about how far away the Faeroe Islands are, I am so glad I did not have any medical problems while I was there.

When I was in Norway, I was not physically strong enough to hike in the mountains. In fact, while I was there, I developed diverticulitis and had to go to the hospital. When I was examined, the physician saw the scar on my chest and wanted to know what my condition had been. When I told him I had a myxoma removed, he was amazed and said,

"In Norway, we only find them in cadavers." Since I was alive to hear that, I felt very lucky.

Needless to say, I enjoyed my visits with family and friends. The mountains were always there, and I enjoyed staring at them. The mountains again inspired me when we went to western Canada later that year. Many people have asked me how long it really takes to recover from open-heart surgery. I know "recover" has different meanings, but it was so frustrating after so many months of recovery and still not being able to return to strenuous hiking.

Early Retirement Plan Offered

Surprisingly, the University offered an early retirement plan, and Ken and I retired on December 31, 2002. We were both 59 years old. We had a great party. I was satisfied because my health was good, and I had had a good career in which I competently taught and performed research until I retired.

Your Enlightenment

When you are recovering from open-heart surgery, concentrate on those activities that you value the most. I felt great delight in walking the trail around our home and seeing wildlife. Everybody does not have the scenery I do (actually, I would enjoy seeing the ocean and mountains even more), but I hope you can enjoy what is available.

I was thrilled when I could swim again. I hope you are able to do physical exercises that make you feel good.

I was excited to be academically competent again, as I had been a professor for 30 years. If you have a profession or an occupation, concentrate on it, but only work at the pace you are able.

Tell others about your surgery so they will be considerate of your limitations. Laugh when you say the wrong word! Do not apologize for it, as you cannot help it.

If you have grandchildren, enjoy playing with them. All I can really say is progress takes time! I am thrilled the medical advances of open-heart surgery were available to me.

3

Three: Beginning My Recovery From A Stroke

Since I was in shock during much of what will be described early in this chapter, I have had to rely on what others have told me. On February 26, 2003, I was swimming alone in our pool. I was accustomed to swimming alone because I was an excellent swimmer. It was cold outside, and there was ice on the patio surrounding our pool. As usual, the water temperature in our pool was 80° F. I was having a good swim. By that time, I could again swim for a half mile each day. I remember floating on my back and observing crystals of ice that formed inside the dome covering the pool. The time was about 10:30 a.m.

After that point, I have few memories. I do not remember climbing the steps out of the pool. I do not remember unfolding the plastic cover and rolling it on the surface of the water. I remember unzipping the opening to the overhead dome and being very cautious because I did not want to fall on the ice on the patio. I remember Ken taking my temperature and that I thought it was a very strange thing for him to do.

Ken had come home and found me searching the house for hot water at about 11:30 a.m. I was furious when I could not find any! I do not remember turning on the whirlpool bathtub, but the tub was full and overflowing through the drain at the top. The water was cold. I had drained all of the water from two hot water tanks.

I had a bad fall somewhere, but only our cats know where that occurred. My injury was slight. I had a large bruise on the inside of my thigh. One kind nurse later said, "Sometimes you never figure out where you hurt yourself."

When Ken found the tub running over, he asked

me what I was doing. Since I had no answer, he knew something was wrong. At first, he thought I was confused due to hypothermia. He then called our internal medicine physician and told him that my temperature was 74° F. The physician said if that were true, I would be dead. Even engineers can make mistakes when they are in a panic! I remember Ken putting me in our sauna to warm me up. Our physician told him to warm me up and bring me to the hospital if I remained confused. I had recently had a physical exam and did not have conditions that would have made him suspicious of my having a stroke. I did not have high blood pressure, and my cholesterol values were normal.

At the Hospital

My confusion continued as Ken drove me to the emergency room of Boone Hospital Center. I shouted the entire way because I thought I could not get my seat belt fastened. In fact, it was on the whole time. I walked into the hospital with Ken close beside me. Ken said I was not walking straight, and he had to pull me by my coat to get me to the door. Since I could not see properly to the left, I kept turning to the right towards the hospital wall. I was unable to understand the receptionist and could not sign my name on the check-in sheet. Ken told them I was confused.

They put me in a bed and took numerous measurements. I did not know what they were doing and was not very cooperative. I complained of being cold, and they wrapped me in hot blankets. I continued to shiver and constantly complained of being cold. In fact, I was not cold, but shivering from shock. I was aware but still very confused.

They took me to the radiology department and performed a CT scan of my head. I remember someone said they were going to bring a neurologist to the emergency ward. They had found two blood clots in my brain. They were of different ages. Apparently, the first one had occurred several days earlier. My only symptom at that time was a bad headache. I was able to give the name of a neurologist I had been seeing for migraine headaches. Although in shock, I amazingly could remember his name. They gave me a chest x-ray, an ECG, and an EEG and admitted me to the hospital.

A Hospital Bed

I was taken to a room in the hospital where I had to be lifted off the gurney because I could not understand what they wanted me to do. A neurologist came to examine me. He asked me to touch my nose with my right hand, which I did. When he then asked me to do the same with my left hand, I responded as before with my right hand. I could look to my right, but not to my left. I could speak, but did not always know what I was saying. I could stand, but not walk. I had no feeling in my left leg. My injuries were greatest immediately following my stroke.

Early the next morning, more tests were done, and by the middle of the morning, I was coherent and could understand and respond to questions. Ken came to see me that morning and was amazed at how normal I looked. My internal medicine physician told me I had had a stroke, and they would find where the clots were coming from. I knew what he said, and I was horrified. I had had open-heart surgery so that I would not have a stroke.

I was immediately put on heparin intravenously. The nurses wanted me to stay in bed, but I wanted to get up whenever I wanted. I thought I could do things I actually could not. I started to move the furniture around. They put an alarm on me, so when I tried to get out of bed, a loud horn went off, and the nurses came and restrained me. They moved my bed in front of the nurses' station so they could see me at all times.

Several months later, a therapist asked me, "Were you the one on the second floor they had to deal with?" Of course, I said "yes," and she grinned at me. I know the nurses were pleased to see me leave that hospital room.

An occupational therapist came by to see me, and they told him to leave me alone because I was not ready for any assistance yet.

A test was ordered to see if my myxoma had grown again and was producing clots. Since I had no other symptoms to explain the stroke, they focused on my prior heart condition. I knew there was a one to two percent chance of the myxoma returning, but no new growth was found. A test to determine my blood-clotting ability was ordered. The results showed that it was very high, and heparin was prescribed to prevent excessive clotting. Certain clotting disorders can be an inherited condition. I informed my brother, and his tested fine.

I could not do anything by myself. Once when three nurses helped me get to the bathroom, I fainted and caused more alarm. They were afraid I had had another stroke, and I was reattached to all of the monitoring instruments so they could monitor my condition. Ken was in my hospital room and had to see all of the instruments connected to me again. I am sure he was terrified, but knew I was in the right place.

Luckily, I was okay, and my fainting had been

caused by my anxiety from all that was going on around me. Since I had always been an independent person, my brain was telling me to do things that my body could not do. An occupational therapist came to assess my condition. He asked me to brush my teeth. I could not hold things well in my left hand, and I tried to squeeze the toothpaste from the tube without removing the cap. I had trouble figuring out logical sequences.

I was prescribed physical therapy to help recover movement in my left arm and leg. Everything moved okay but not at the right time or with enough strength. I have realized how fortunate I was that I did not have any paralysis. I was to have occupational therapy so I could re-learn common tasks we do every day. I also needed speech therapy, which confused me because my speech was fine. I later learned the nature of speech therapy and why it was beneficial to my recovery.

The Kind of Stroke I Had

After all the tests, it was found I had an embolism,

or a traveling blood clot, in the right side of my brain in the parietal lobe. Each side of the brain is served by different blood vessels. Those in the area of the clot fed the tissue controlling my left side, causing my left side to be affected. Strokes usually damage only one side of the body. Symptoms appear on the side of the body opposite the damaged side of the brain. Some of my brain cells died from a lack of blood. My neurologist showed this to me months later when we studied my brain scan. I prefer to say that some of my brain cells were "stunned."

The Inpatient Rehabilitation Unit

I was moved to the inpatient rehabilitation unit, and I remember the nurse saying, "You are lucky we have room, because sometimes all the beds are full." Due to the shortage of patients, I did not have another patient in my room for the entire length of my visit. I went to the rehab unit in a wheelchair, with the heparin meter on a cart with wheels trailing behind me. This "thing" was attached to a tube in my arm, and I started referring to my portable IV pole as "George." By this time, I was able to answer some questions about my age, degrees I had, and the name of the hospital. I still could not put my left finger on my nose.

I was given a bed and a very kind nurse assured me she would be taking care of me. They gave me a buzzer and told me to use it whenever I needed anything. I was not to go anywhere without their help. The nurses took care of my general health and daily needs whenever I was not in therapy. They pushed me to do things on my own as soon as I could. At first, I stayed in bed most of the time. I got in the habit of eating my meals in bed. For my meals, they gave me a card to indicate what I wanted for breakfast (7 a.m.), lunch (noon), and dinner (5 p.m.). For several days, I was not capable of completing this card. As I cannot eat beef, I had to be very careful about my selections. Every slip that came with the meals indicated "no beef." Ken brought in my special decaf tea, which the nurses made for me. Ken also brought in the

fiber-rich cereal I enjoy. As soon as I could sit in a chair, the nurse made me get out of bed to eat. She said, "It is not normal to eat in bed."
My one-month long stay in the inpatient rehabilitation unit had begun.

Setting Your Pace in an Inpatient Rehabilitation Unit

Prior to my stroke, I did not know what a rehabilitation unit was. Neither I nor my friends or family had ever been in one. A neurologist was responsible for the unit. A nurse was in charge of my everyday care. Along with Ken, she interviewed me when I was admitted to the unit. She asked me many demeaning questions, such as, "What is the name of this hospital?" I answered correctly, but a few days earlier, I would not have known. The neurologist frequently asked the same question, which I soon learned was one of the techniques used to assess my progress. At one point, I was tempted to give him the wrong name of the hospital. But I did not because I did not want to suffer the consequences.

Therapists visited the rehab unit on a regular basis. The neurologist directed the care I received from the occupational, physical, recreational, and speech therapists. The therapists had a schedule for my rehabilitation exercises, and held a meeting every Thursday afternoon to discuss the progress of their patients.

The nurses had a schedule for waking me, serving meals, giving me showers, and attending to my "call" button. Visiting hours were from 8 a.m. to 8 p.m. I did not like being on a routine, but I soon realized that was the only way the unit could be run effectively. I would have preferred to eat when I wanted to, wake up when I was ready to, and have showers when I needed them. I had no choice but to accept what they thought would help me.

I had a very pleasant experience during my first week in the unit after I was given a shower. Showers were allowed only every other day, and I had to wait my turn. They were decided by even and odd hospital room numbers.

Giving me a shower was not an easy process. The

shower was easy to get in and out of, and the shower head had flexible control. However, I initially was not capable of setting the correct water temperature and could not control the shower head. I had trouble figuring out what part of my body to wash first. I got shampoo in my eyes. The nurses were alarmed because my eyes turned red. My shower head went everywhere, including the floor beside the tub. I soon learned why showers were rationed—because they took too much labor. It was then I realized how important smells were to me. Ken had brought in my shampoo and conditioner. I thoroughly enjoyed being able to smell my shampoo. I also had the same pleasant experience when Ken brought in my personal deodorant. When you are in a hospital, it can be comforting to bring in your own toiletries. Familiarity makes a great difference. After a shower, I thought I could more easily accept the orders I was being given.

After I showered, the nurses had to ensure I was fully dry and then blow-dry my hair. It would be several weeks before I could do this task by myself.

Total Devastation

I was devastated about being in the rehab unit. Having had a myxoma removed so I would not have a stroke, and then having one anyway, made me furious. My internal medicine physician asked if I needed something for depression, but I refused. He said, "Let me know if you change your mind and let me know before your depression gets too bad. You probably do not believe this now, but one day you will be scrambling to get out of here." He asked Ken if he needed depression medication. Ken said he was getting along okay. I felt lucky I had been to my physician enough times that he knew me. Having a physician who knew me helped my emotional recovery. I never took any medicine for depression. I just knew I could cope with whatever happened.

My physicians made frequent trips to see me. I had very congenial relationships with them. When I had a physical problem, the nurse called my internal medicine physician. As my heparin dosage was closely monitored, he explained the role of the drug, and adjusted the dosage as necessary. My neurologist was responsible for the medications that affected my brain. He checked my reflexes and showed delight when I could place my left finger to my nose. Frequently, both my neurologist and internal medicine physician came to see me when I was attempting to put on my make-up. This was unusual because not many patients on that unit had insisted on wearing make-up. They laughed with me as it became easier. We discussed my treatment, and they knew I wanted to completely recover as soon as possible.

I wanted to be involved in my recovery. When I told my physician I had the opportunity to be a member of an international committee for food technology, he encouraged me. He reassured me that if I kept up the hard work, I would be able to accept this opportunity, as I would not have to travel to a meeting until July 2003. That greatly helped my psychological state.

How I Got Around My Hospital Room

Initially, I used a wheelchair. Getting around with my portable IV pole, "George," beside me was very awkward at first. Later, I was taught to use a walker. Again, "George" was beside me. As I had little feeling in my left leg, I could easily fall. I was paranoid about being safe. Learning to use a walker was tricky. I was given complete instructions about how to use it. My father-in-law was in a retirement home where he used one, and I often thought of him as I moved about my room. Walkers look so easy when you see someone else using one, but I assure you they are not. Having a walker was certainly easier then being confined to a wheelchair, as I had increased mobility. By the end of my stay, I could walk around the room without any support.

During a restless night in the rehabilitation unit, a male nurse asked me if he could help me. I told him I was having difficulty putting on my bra. I decided a sports bra would be better for me, and I knew I had two at home. I asked the nurse to call Ken and ask him to bring in my sports bra. He refused because it was 4 a.m. So, at 7 a.m., I called Ken, and he brought them in later that morning. As it turned out, they were even harder to put on than my regular bra. Why do I do most of my serious thinking in the middle of the night?

Learning to Read Again

One Sunday when no therapists were in the hospital, the nurse on duty found me trying to read, and observed my frustration. She asked, "Do you want me to show you how to read?" I accepted her help. She was hesitant, because that was not one of her nursing functions.

She started out by saying, "This is what I have observed from the therapists teaching others." She instructed me to draw a vertical line along the margin on the left side of the page with a thick marker. Then, she took a blank piece of paper and placed it under the words. My vision was good, but I did not have enough attention span to read from left to right and stay on the same line. Using her technique, I was able to see the left-hand side of the page. By having blank paper under each line, I did not skip around and was able to focus. I slowly read with her. I used this technique for the next three weeks.

I truly appreciated her response to my frustration. Being able to read boosted my morale. That was one less thing I had to re-learn.

Each time Ken came to visit, he straightened my glasses because I was not capable of placing them correctly above my left ear. He brought the mail and papers I normally read each day. He brought *The Wall Street Journal* and *Foreign Affairs*. It was important to me to see that they were available.

One day when Ken brought *The Wall Street Journal,* some of my colleagues were pictured on the front page. I had been with them in October 2002, at a conference in California, where they were discussing the potential of having a war, talking about what would later become known as Operation Iraqi Freedom. My food science associates were discussing how food was going to be delivered to Iraq. So, I wanted to read this paper! I followed the instructions the nurse had given me and read the first page. The text then said: continued on page 22, column 6. That was the hardest part for me, as I had to find page 22 and figure out where column 6 was. I was finally able to read my story.

At that point, I was elated! I shared my success with everyone. I wonder what any of my food science colleagues would have thought if they knew what a challenge they gave me by reporting to the *Wall Street Journal*. After that success, reading was much easier for me. Losing my ability to read was a terrible loss, especially when my academic life had depended on it.

Working with Therapists

All of the therapists helping me had their own specialties. At first, I was kind of like a robot following their directions. I use the term "robot" because that was how I was instructed to act. I felt like I had no other option but to follow along with the strategy they had designed for me, which was an uncomfortable concept.

I had a great deal of fear of the unknown. I wanted to know when I would be able to dress myself, when I could walk without support, and what came next in my rehabilitation. So, I started asking these questions. All of the answers they gave me included the phrase, "all strokes are different." I hated hearing that statement because I wanted concrete answers. Of course, none were available. So, I tried to patiently follow their directions because I assumed they were taking good care of me.

Occupational Therapists

Occupational therapy uses activities of everyday living to help patients with physical and mental disabilities achieve maximum functioning at home and at work. Occupational therapy benefits people of all ages, from infants to the elderly, and can improve function whether the disability results from birth defect, accident, disease, aging, or drug or alcohol abuse. Occupational therapy is geared to the function and interests of the patient. Occupational therapists also work with people with mental and emotional problems, such as depression or anxiety. I worked with several occupational therapists.

An occupational therapist was the first therapist to see me. Occupational therapy sounds like training for a job, but I found out that it is lot more. It includes the everyday things you have to do to be "on your own." I did not have to wear hospital gowns after the second day, since Ken had brought in my normal clothes and toiletries from home. I wore jogging suits during the day and nightgowns at night. Being in my own clothes gave me a good feeling. My occupational therapist asked, "Where do you normally get dressed?" She wanted to know if I got dressed while I was standing or sitting. I did not know. She laid out my clothes for me "in order." I needed complete instructions. I had to learn to put my underwear on before my sweatpants. I had to learn to put my clothes on right side out. All the time I was in the hospital, she had to hook my bra in the back. I had to learn to put on both of my socks before she put on my jogging shoes. I learned how many ways a shirt with four holes can be put on wrong. I learned the label in the neck tells you front from back.

At the end of the month, I was finally able to tie my shoes without help. It took me two months before I could easily tie a double knot. There were a few things said to me to which I objected. People said, "You know that children also have trouble learning to tie their shoes." I was not a child, and I did not like being referred to as one. But, of course, I had to re-learn things as if I were a child again. It is not as frustrating for children because they are learning tasks for the first time.

Fortunately, your brain can re-learn what it has lost. I struggled. I lost my temper with Ken when he said, "That is so simple even children can do it." I rarely lose my temper, so this was a different experience. I knew he meant it in kindness, but those statements were awfully hard to hear.

Behind my temper was the realization that I would eventually accomplish what I could not do now. I would show them I could dress myself and perform any other challenges they demanded. When I had accomplished those challenges, then I thought I would accept their genuine encouragement because it was real, and I would know it was said with all sincerity.

When I went to the bathroom, I said I did not need help. I thought I would have no problem, as there was a buzzer in there in case I needed help. During my first solo visit, I was standing with the help of a walker and "George" in front of the toilet seat. I stood there, not knowing whether to pull my sweatpants up or down. Finally I realized I should pull them down and sit on the cold toilet seat. I also had to struggle to remember to pull my underwear down. So, from then on, "A Cold Toilet Seat" was my motto. Feeling so foolish, I never told anyone in the hospital about my initial situation. I hated it every day when a nurse asked me if I had a bowel movement that day, but I had to answer her.

The therapists were always encouraging me, telling me I got better by the day, by the week, and by the month. It was hard for me to believe the therapists actually saw I was really improving. Getting dressed was such a demeaning task that I wrongly thought I did not need to be encouraged. I thought I was improving as fast as I could. The occupational therapist was correct in giving me encouragement. I often wondered, was it genuine? Should I believe her? I had to believe the rigorous atmosphere I was in would help me. I had to trust in others' knowledge. All I could do was appreciate what I had. Trusting in the hospital staff became easier with my progress.

The occupational therapist asked me, "Do you always wear makeup?" I said, "Yes!" Too many bad things had happened to me, so why should anyone see me looking even worse? So, from then on, she gave me extra time to let me figure out how to put on my make-up. I did not have much feeling on my left side. I was not paralyzed, but I felt numb, a condition called apraxia. At first, I could not open the containers for my foundation, powder, blush, or eye shadow. She recommended I be consistent, putting liquid foundation on both the left and right sides of my face.

I frequently "lost" things. A nurse laughed and said, "When you lose anything, just look in your left hand." It was usually there. The one thing I could do perfectly was put on mascara! I never made a mistake or stuck myself in the eye. At that point, I could not yet read, but I could put on mascara. I cannot explain this. I was soon able to open the containers alone, and became faster at putting on make-up.

Eating in the Dining Room

Another assignment the occupational therapists had was to see if I needed any help eating. I was assigned to eat in the dining room every Monday. Everyone else on the unit was much older than I, and had serious problems with eating. I remember those meals with shudders. I observed how badly they ate and heard their conversations.

They were talking about what it was like to farm in the 1940's. They needed a great deal of assistance with eating. I needed no help!

However, the therapist said I was eating the wrong way. Actually, I used the British system; using both my knife and fork. I insisted I was eating correctly. I showed her how I could pick up a green pea from my plate, and she stopped insisting I change. I learned to eat that way when I was six years old, and nobody was going to change me.

Another part of having me eat in the dining room was to help my "sociability." As I had lots of visitors with whom I enjoyed talking, that was not necessary in my mind. Fortunately, when Operation Iraqi Freedom started, I was glued to my television, and the nurses gave me a reprieve from eating in the dining room.

When Ken and I had our initial discussion with an occupational therapist, she asked me what my hobbies were. I said I cooked and gardened. Because their purpose was to help me become competent at home, they arranged activities around cooking and gardening. I went along with their activities, but they proved to be very frustrating.

Cooking Class

As hardly anybody cooks extensively today, the occupational therapist was not an accomplished cook. I did not ask, but I am sure learning to cook was not part of her degree program. Compared to my organized, large kitchen at home, the hospital kitchen was a joke, however I tried to be cooperative. The therapist was paranoid about my safety. She did not want me to burn anything or cut myself. I did not want to be in that kitchen. I felt I exerted a great deal of patience just being in that kitchen.

As a food scientist, being able to cook was much more than a hobby. Previously, I could bake any recipe for brownies, in any size of pan, from 8x8 inch square to a hotel-size pan. All I needed was a recipe. I certainly would not have used brownies in a box with instructions. I had never bought boxes of brownies that had step 1, step 2, and step 3 on the package. Now, I was given a box of brownie mix in an unfamiliar kitchen. I did not know how to make the pan stick-free, once I found a pan. I did not know how to measure the correct amount of water, once I had located a measuring cup. My occupational therapist hovered over me so I would do things correctly. When I made the brownies, I was in a wheelchair and "George" was also in the kitchen. I almost forgot to put the eggs in because I had to find them in the refrigerator. I did not have a clue about how to turn on the oven or set the timer, because those actions involved numbers.

My emotional state was precarious because I knew how to bake brownies, but I was totally incapable that day. I certainly wondered if I would be able to cook again. Being hovered over did not help my state of mind. Any encouragement I received on that day was not appreciated. A nurse told me they ate my brownies at the nurse's station, and I just laughed. My thought was, "poor you."

The next class came three weeks later, closer to the end of my stay. It was to involve "stir-fry," and I was dreading it. My occupational therapist brought in a frozen package of stir-fry ingredients and some chicken that I was directed to cut up. The knives were so dull that I just made a mess. All they had to cook stir-fry "in" was a large frying pan. My therapist had dropped the soy sauce in the parking lot, and she told me we could substitute salt. I guess by that time I was beginning to sound like a food scientist. I said, "No way can we make that substitution." I told her to go to the hospital kitchen and ask for some soy sauce, and she did. We started to cook everything, and I told her when it was ready. She argued with me because she did not want the vegetables to be crisp. We finished cooking and ate our stir-fry. My therapist and I clearly had different tastes. She asked me, "What do you cook?" I replied, "Everything," which was a foreign concept to her. I took great delight in having those exercises over.

After eating what we had prepared, my therapist

said, "Everything went very well in the kitchen today." I did not agree, but I gave her a courteous smile. I was happy I would never have to be in that kitchen again! I did not complain about her "lack of abilities." Perhaps other patients who did not have my experience would perform with her in a more positive manner. Deep down, I wanted her to say, "You are a food scientist, so you must be more qualified than I."

I worried that I would never be able to function as a food scientist again. This was a very hard concept for me to bear. Would I be able to have parties for fifty friends and do the catering? Would I be able to answer questions everyone always asked me about food and nutrition? I had too many unknowns. I had spent my professional life being first a dietitian and then a food scientist. I did not even know how much my academic memory would be affected. Would I be able to answer questions about food chemistry, food microbiology, food physics, and food engineering? My only consolation was I knew I had retired.

Gardening In My Red Pajamas

Because I liked to garden, my therapist told me one day she had brought pansies to the hospital. We had to plant them that day, as rain was forecast for late that afternoon. That was the day before I was going to have a colonoscopy, and I was wearing my red pajamas so I could get my pants off in a hurry if necessary. Although I argued, we went to a mini-garden outside the hospital where nobody could see us. First, I had to figure out how to get the pansies out of the container. Then, I had to dig the dirt and plant them fourteen inches apart, which was a challenge for me to measure. Luckily, the rain started late in the afternoon, and we had to go inside. I was told I should watch for rain during the next week. I should water them if it did not rain. Fortunately, it rained torrents. During our efforts, she said things that sounded silly to me like, "When you plant, make sure you put plants on both the right and left side of the garden." I hadn't realized I was making mistakes while I was working with her.

Looking back on these two experiences, I did them only because I was directed. They seemed like such trivial efforts to cook and garden. I was impatient, and as it turned out, it took me a long time before I was able to do those things well. I guess I felt that if I did them, I would give the therapist a good impression of me. I thought that was necessary because everything else she did for me had really helped. She was trying to get me to realize that mastering those silly lessons would help me to cook and garden at home.

Physical Therapists

A physical therapist uses scientific physical procedures to treat patients with a disability, disease, or injury to help them achieve and maintain functional rehabilitation and to prevent malfunction or deformity. Treatments are individually designed to hasten convalescence and help patients' comfort and well-being. Physical therapy is prescribed for patients with varied orthopedic, neurological, vascular, and respiratory conditions. Several physical therapists were employed in my rehabilitation center. Several of them told me that they enjoyed their profession because they could easily see patients improve. In the U.S., physical therapists have three types of training: a certificate program, a Bachelor of Science program, and a Master of Science program. The Council on Medical Education, in collaboration with the American Physical Therapy Association, provides therapy education and practice. Licensing or registration is required in almost all states.

After I was dressed and had my make-up on, a physical therapist was scheduled to help me every day. So, I wondered, "Will a physical therapist let me walk on my own?" I had no clue. I just had to do as she suggested. My thoughts were numerous: what if I have to spend the rest of my life in a wheelchair? I knew we had built our home in case either of us needed wheelchairs. We even had a permanent ramp from our car court to our kitchen. What if I always had to use a walker?

What if I always had to use a cane? Either device would prevent me from vigorous hiking. Would I be strong enough to swim? I silently had all of these questions at the start of my physical therapy sessions. I knew not to ask these questions because I would get my standard answer that "all strokes are different."

Being in "good" physical shape, I gained a great deal from physical therapy. Although I was not paralyzed, particular effort was spent working to regain strength and balance on my left side. At first, a physical therapist lifted me out of my wheelchair and strapped me to her so I would not fall. Being strapped to someone is not a reassuring experience. I walked down the hallway with "George" on wheels beside me. She noted how far I walked. I walked several yards the first day before I became too tired and had to go back to my room. The therapist had always cautioned me to stop when I got too tired, so I was helped back to bed and waited for the next therapist. When I was able to walk the complete length of the hallway, the physical therapist wheeled me to the gym where I had more space to walk.

Most of the other patients in the gym were recovering from knee replacement surgery. They were suffering! Seeing them struggle when I was walking with no pain made me realize I was better off than I thought. In the gym, I had to learn how to climb up and down three wooden stairs. Initially, I was terrified. Going up the stairs was easier than coming down. I was safe because I always had a strap attached to my physical therapist. Many of the exercises helped me with balance. My left side was very weak and I tried to compensate by using my right side. The therapist had to keep stopping me from compensating.

Sometimes both occupational and physical therapists were with me. They threw balls for me to catch and observed how I "caught" them and was able to "return" them. At this time, my balance was good enough I did not need to have a strap. Finally, I was able to progress further. I was instructed to walk up and down hospital stairs. As it got warmer,

I was able to walk outside. Going outside gave me a wonderful feeling. I had to walk up and down the sidewalks and on uneven grass surfaces, always on hospital grounds. I often wondered if some of my friends or colleagues had driven by the hospital and seen me strapped to the physical therapist.

The therapists also came up with games that would help in rehabilitation. One day, they made me a "waitress," and I had to show how I could hold a tray of plastic cups in my left hand. I dropped most of them. At first, I spilled a lot of water. Next, to help my attention span, they placed 20 cups around the gym in high places to see if I could find them. On my last day of physical therapy, both the occupational and physical therapists threw balls with me outdoors. I was beginning to feel my freedom.

I gained many skills from physical therapy. It was at this time that my internal medicine physician prescribed Coumadin instead of heparin. I was elated, as "George" was finally retired and I had more freedom. I learned to walk, initially with a strap, and then alone. My balance became much better. I can never say that I always had perfect balance throughout my life. When my therapist threw balls to me, and I almost fell, she said, "You saved yourself well." I could walk on rough surfaces. I was cautioned to take care at curbs. It would have been good if my physical therapist knew what my balance was before I had a stroke, but that was not possible.

I made a lot of improvements, and by the time I was discharged, I could receive and throw balls outdoors. I developed a good sense of accomplishment through physical therapy. I was keenly aware of my difficulties on my left side, and I knew I just had to adjust. Having a sense of accomplishment was extremely important to me. **I gathered assurance that I could function reasonably well with my limitations.**

I knew I could walk alone without falling. I knew I had to be careful on bumpy surfaces. I knew my balance was acceptable, as long as I did not exert myself. There was no way I was ever going to throw balls! I had not done that before I had a stroke. I knew I would always need to be cautious when I walked, taking care where my feet were stepping. Most importantly, I knew I could handle my physical state. I hoped I would not develop a limp, but if I did, limping would be much better than being confined to a walker, and I would concentrate on exercising my leg as much as possible.

Recreational Therapists

As I have never played "games" for fun, I was frustrated with recreational therapy. I had to do simple word puzzles and play games like dominoes, which all seemed boring to me. Since then, I have realized these games were to exercise my brain, not for entertainment. Later, at home, I did many of these exercises. I can imagine others in the ward loved to do this therapy, such as learning to play bridge again. Instead, I wanted to do something more productive that would help me become more competent. I frequently said I wanted to "get competent." That was, in fact, a ridiculous term for me to use. I would never able to become as competent as I had been before.

I could tell I did not please the recreational therapist very much. My attitude toward her was not as kind as it should have been, because I felt other activities would help me more.

Several times, she wanted me to go to the lobby and find my own way back to my hospital bed. That was a difficult task. It took me four weeks of practice in therapy sessions to accomplish it.

Speech Therapists

Speech is a learned system of communication requiring the coordination of voice, articulation, and language skills. In a broad sense, speech is synonymous with language. Speech therapists have been trained to diagnose and treat the various disorders of speech, language, and voice. Physical, neurological, or psychological conditions are frequently related to a speech disorder. The speech therapist often works as a member of a team that includes a neurologist, psychiatrist, and psychological social worker.

Speech therapists have Bachelor of Science and Master of Science degrees in speech pathology. They are responsible for teaching a speech-impaired person to think appropriately in verbal terms and to exercise control over speech disorders by emotional influences. When patients lose their ability to perform mathematics and think logically, it becomes the speech therapists' role to help them. Several speech therapists were employed in my rehabilitation unit. I told them frequently that they had the wrong term for their profession, as they did much more than handle speech and language concerns. They usually grinned and said, "That's how it is."

Since I did not have any speech problems, I was confused when I was told I needed speech therapy. I quickly learned speech therapists do much more than help people with their speaking ability. Another name for their profession could be cognitive therapist, but psychologists have trouble with that term.

Ken was with me for my first session with the speech therapist. She asked me many questions that reminded me of those asked my father-in-law when he was assessed for Alzheimer's disease. I told her so, and she assured me she had other reasons. She asked me a lot of questions about my feelings and my attitude, and I found that her purpose was to diagnose depression. I was not depressed. She asked Ken if I always used the same manner and tone. He said, "Yes, she is as direct and persistent as usual." The therapist said she was trying to determine whether my personality had changed. Some people have drastic changes in personality after having a stroke. In effect, they become different people. Luckily, my personality was still "me."

An area of my brain that was affected was the math/logic area. The therapist brought me arithmetic problems. I could not count things, and I had trouble with my attention span. I could not add 1+1=2. When she gave me a list of math questions to do, I was not consistent when I went down the list. I would start at the top and miss some lines or some of the questions on a line. Many times I would say, "I can't do it" or "I don't care." At the end of the session, she would "grade" me. I was upset at being graded on such simple things.

One time, the therapist stopped me because, by the look on my face, she knew I was going to tell her I had a Ph.D. I did not need any self-pity. I remember telling my second cousins, who were in middle school, I had zero percent correct on my homework. I showed them the math I could not do. Of course, they laughed. I do not know what they really thought! Here I was lying in bed, doing homework they could easily do, and I was a total failure.

Initially, I hated visits by the speech therapist. When she tried to help me, my brain "ached" after thirty minutes. Of course, my brain was not aching, but the effort I was making taxed my abilities. I wanted to go home and stroke a cat. Because that was not possible, I had to contemplate my current situation. I realized numbers are totally involved with one's life. I needed to use them to do things such as read the clock, make financial decisions, read TV and airline schedules, find page numbers in a book or magazine, find call numbers in a library, and understand political polls. So I had to proceed! I did not think I would be returning to my previous abilities for doing statistics. I guess I had the attitude that I was retired, and that part of my life was behind me.

The speech therapist could not have been more patient. She realized when I did not care, and she knew how to be persistent with me. She never told me about my inabilities. I had to figure out for myself how mathematical and logistical inefficiencies would affect my life. As I was lying in bed dreading the therapist's next visit, I felt I was in a strange situation. I knew I eventually had to learn to do math, but I was not capable of doing even simple tasks. Knowing you cannot do something, and knowing you should know how to do it, is a real dilemma. My dilemma was even worse because of the fact that I once excelled at math and could always make logical decisions. Finally, my speech therapist observed I had reached the point where I wanted to improve.

We progressed from being able to add and subtract two digits, then three digits. It took ages for me to understand how to carry numbers. Of course, I could not use a calculator in the hospital. Then I had to learn how to multiply and divide. She gave me homework that was due the next day. On one occasion, I did a terrible job, giving all the wrong answers. In response to my frustration, the therapist said, "You cannot do this because you have had a stroke." It took awhile for me to realize why I was so incompetent. When she left my room, I heard her say to one nurse, "We made some progress today."

One exercise she gave me was about "sales." I always buy clothes "on sale." The exercise was to buy a suit. They were "on sale." The percentages discounted and the tagged sale prices were different. My task was to come up with the best choice. This question was important to me, as that is how

I buy clothes, so I dreamt about it that night and shared the dream with my speech therapist the next morning. Apparently, it was discussed at their weekly group meeting with the neurologist and the question was raised whether they were working me too hard. I said, "No, I always work at night." I do my best thinking in the middle of the night. I wrote my Ph.D. dissertation by thinking in the middle of the night. I urged them to keep pushing me.

The speech therapist started to give me simple word problems. By that time, I started to refer to her as "my professor." When she gave me word problems to solve, she called this "functional" math. I enjoyed trying to solve them, especially when I had to do multiple steps to get the correct answer. She would give me one set of problems, and I would try to do them with her guidance. I could only get a few correct, and the next day, she would bring the same problems, and try again. Again, I would make errors.

I objected to this approach because, in my academic life, I had complex problems to solve, and I correctly solved them. I did not receive the same solved problems to do again! However, the speech therapist gave me the same problems again and again until I could solve them. I think my frustration level hindered how well I could solve them.

It is hard to summarize what I learned from speech therapy. I certainly did not take notes when I could easily add 1 + 2 = 3 or readily subtract 8 from 12, but I did learn other basic math tasks. I could only do them if I thought about them carefully. I could not multiply 7 x 7 and get a rapid answer of 49. From that point on, I knew my thinking process was slow. Needless to say, I made much progress in the unit, especially when my attitude toward math became much more positive.

I realized I would always be able to use calculators at a later date, but a calculator is just a small part of how I was going to use math on a functional basis. How would I determine how much dry cat food to give our cats, based on their weight and the amount of food they required per pound? How would I count the antibiotic pills to give to our cats? And, on a human side, could I calculate the weight Ken and I had to lose or gain to stay within our ideal weight ranges? Could I understand the outdoor temperature and dress appropriately? Could I understand my calendar so I could put appointments on correct dates and at the correct time? Would I be able to recognize an airplane flight at the correct gate and arrival or departure times?

When I left the inpatient rehabilitation unit, I did not know the answers to these questions. At that time, I could list hundreds of math and logistical questions I was not certain I would know. I was terrified! I assumed I had made some progress, but would I make more improvements? I certainly knew, at that point, that my thinking process had rapidly deteriorated. Would my thinking process get even slower, or would it improve? When I asked these questions to everyone, I got the standard answer, "all strokes are different." So, my improvement was up to me!

I had to be persistent and take further speech

therapy if it became available to me. Having my last inpatient speech therapy session was a terrible experience for me. I clearly was not "functional." I wanted "my professor" to teach me more. I had to realize she had done all she could with me. The speech therapist had transformed me from a person who was indifferent to a person who cared to learn. As a professor, that was something I always wanted to do with my students. Sometimes I was successful; sometimes I failed. I knew if students were excited about food science, their attitudes usually made them excel, given that my lectures would enliven them. So I left the rehabilitation unit knowing I needed to learn much more from the speech therapist.

I used to tell friends I could not do math. Often they would say, "That is what calculators are for. You can always use one." I knew math was much more than handling the simple tasks. However, I did not argue with their simplicity. **I guess I understood the rest of my life would involve math. I was scared!**

A Terrible Party With A Good Ending

Therapists did many positive things for me, but I got off to a rough start. I want to relate this negative experience to you because it ultimately had a very positive result. I left the inpatient rehabilitation ward much stronger because of this incident.

When I had been on the inpatient rehabilitation unit for only a few days, I was invited to a "party" in the gym. The purpose of the occasion was a group of patients were being discharged from the unit, and a party had been planned to celebrate the success they had achieved. "George" and I were wheeled to the gym. I was parked along a wall for a while as the other patients arrived. As I have explained, I was 59 years old and the other patients were much older. My initial reaction was that I was sitting there with "those old folks." I was confined to my wheelchair, and "George" was beside me, giving me heparin intravenously. The therapists had arranged activities for us. After a considerable wait, we were instructed to play horseshoes. I had never played horseshoes before, and although I hated playing games, I went along with it. "George" and I began to throw horseshoes. When I won the game, my reaction was, "So what?" Next, we played bingo, and I won again. So again, what did this matter to me? Next, our task was to wrap up t-shirts the hospital was going to give the patients who were being released from the unit. I could not wrap a parcel. Next, "George" and I were wheeled into the kitchen, and I was told to make coffee. I did not know how the coffee pot worked, and I certainly could not count how many tablespoons of coffee grounds I needed. The therapists finally had to make the coffee.

Fortunately, Ken was waiting for me in my hospital room when I returned and I was crying. When I explained the party scene to him, he said, "Complain about it." So the next morning, when my neurologist came for a visit, I told him the therapists were not working me hard enough. He explained that patients could not improve before they were ready. I agreed with him.

The next day when Ken asked the neurologist about my condition, he said, "I have never had a patient complain they were not given enough work to do. I left instructions to the staff to challenge her." Thereafter, when therapists checked my chart, they saw the instructions that told them to "challenge me." They followed these instructions. When I left the inpatient unit, and I could walk out on my own, the social worker said to me, "I am glad you spoke your mind; most people do not say anything." I never had to participate in a group function again while I was in the unit.

I spent a lot of time in the unit with only thinking to do. One day, a nurse asked me, "What are you thinking about?" At that time, I was remembering a trip I had taken in October and November 2002. I had gone to a professional meeting, and then had met relatives at Newport Beach, California. I was remembering how much I enjoyed being on the ocean. Whenever I am there, I usually tell them, "This is the greatest place to be."

Next, I went to my hometown of Vancouver. Those of you who visit Canada know that the trees in the eastern part of Canada have leaves that turn brilliant colors. However, on the West Coast, the leaves are not nearly as colorful. When our plane was descending into the Vancouver airport, I observed this was not the case that fall. The colorful leaves were outstanding. The fall had been very dry. My friends and I took great pleasure in walking through the dried leaves. When we walked through Stanley Park (I hope you have seen this wonderful location), a huge maple leaf floated down before us under the Lions Gate Bridge. In my mind, I am probably exaggerating its size, but it is a leaf I will always remember.

I answered the nurse by telling her about my recent travels. She appreciated my pleasure and said, "It is good you have many good times to talk about. Many patients come in here and are so sad they did not visit the places they wanted to see when they were able, and now they are just sad for the opportunities they missed."

Visitors Sure Make A Difference

I had many caring family members and friends come to visit me in the rehabilitation unit. I was lying in bed and my speech was good. Apparently, I tried not to exhibit any "stroke characteristics." That was a silly thing to do, as the effects of having a stroke are much worse than a friend's first impression.

A retirement party had been scheduled for me on the first of March. Obviously, I was not able to go. A friend gave me a wonderful pillow with a cotton flannel cover, which I used throughout my stay, as I soon realized that hospital pillows were terrible! The visitors I remember most were those who told me something about themselves. I was just lying there, so being told an event in their lives was important to me. Their experiences gave me something more to think about. When they hesitated about something to say, I asked them about their children, grandchildren, dogs or cats. As I am a cat lover, I was given a cat pillow for our cat room. Friends who came in and said prayers with me were wonderful!

I appreciated receiving flowers and baskets of fruit, and people who came in laughing and saying "Look at you!" They were fun because I could laugh with them!

I had to laugh at a ridiculous thing that happened. I recently asked a friend how I was when she came to see me in the inpatient rehabilitation unit. She visited after I had been there for about ten days. She said I was euphoric, and that I kept saying I was glad to be alive. I had laughed with her, and she told me she left my room with a really good feeling about how I was going to improve. I guess going from being devastated to euphoric did not take me very long. Everyone says I always had a positive attitude, and I never got depressed. Clearly, I was self-determined and strong-willed.

Another friend who is an occupational therapist frequently came in to check on my progress. She gave no advice, but I could tell she was quietly assessing my progress.

When I got a zero percent on my math, I shared it

with my visitors! I soon realized it was important to be honest about the "slow" progress I thought I was making. Many friends said they sensed losing my ability to do math made me feel distraught, and I felt a huge sense of loss because it deterred from my independent state.

Often, I was confused, and thought "Why me?" to myself, but I constantly exhibited a sense of optimism to others. I knew I must rely on others for their knowledge, including physicians, neurologists, nurses, and therapists. When I asked a friend who came to visit at the end of my stay in the inpatient unit how I was, he said I was eager to go home! I had had enough of being in a regimented situation, which showed them I had made a great deal of progress.

Some friends found it too hard to visit because they were afraid of the effects of my stroke, and instead sent flowers. When I called to say "thank you" (once I had mastered the telephone), they were excited to hear my voice and were glad I could speak clearly. I certainly understood their reaction and believe I would have had a similar reaction. Strokes do many terrible things to so many people. I continue to be pleased I had a "light" stroke, whatever that means.

Children And Therapy Dogs

Visits from children were very special. They could not understand why I could not do the math they were learning to do in middle school. Some brought me dominoes because they heard a recreational therapist had said I should learn how to play that game. I believed it was important for children to see me, especially my second cousins, who could possibly see me totally recover. They had only known older people who did not recover from a stroke. I hoped that would give them a positive perspective when they heard someone had suffered a stroke.

On Sundays, therapy dogs were brought in to visit patients. They were remarkable and extremely well behaved. A wonderful black Labrador was wearing a white tie and white cuffs! All the dogs had gone through therapy training. They were a delight! If you enjoy dogs they have been trained well, they make terrific visitors. I was always asked if I would like them to come into my room. I was happy to welcome them.

I found that short, frequent visits were more enjoyable than long visits. I appreciated when friends expressed their goal to help, and verbalized that this was a new experience for them, too. I'm sure Ken appreciated our friends' thoughtful gestures toward him as well.

Here is what I valued most about my visitors: they showed me concern and monitored my progress, they shared news about friends and the community with me, they made me laugh, they shared some events with me about their personal lives, and they were always positive. I am determined to master these skills for being a good hospital visitor.

Your Enlightenment

This section should probably start by saying, "Get to the hospital as soon as possible." However, in my case, that was Ken's job, as I was in total shock. Instead, I am going to concentrate on life in the rehabilitation unit.

Be as independent as you are allowed to be in the unit. Wear what you want to wear. Comfortable clothes without zippers are the best. Make sure you have good shoes so you will not slip. Struggle with make-up if that is important to you. Follow the advice given to you by your therapists. Do not refuse to do anything you are physically and mentally capable of doing. Do everything possible not to fall. When it is justified, speak to your neurologist about your treatment plan.

You will eventually see progress. In other words, take all the advice offered to you. Laugh when you can and do everything you can to be a good patient. You will improve, slowly at first, and then more rapidly. You will leave with the knowledge that you are able to accept further challenges at home.

4

Four: Adjusting To My Different Life At Home

Before being discharged, an occupational and physical therapist drove me home for an in-home inspection. I drew them a map so they could find their way. As we live in the country, I had drawn many maps, so I thought it would be easy. However, it was an effort to draw. Once out on the roads, I could give them good directions.

I appreciated the fact that they wanted an in-depth tour of our home. They commented that many houses are much more crowded than ours. Without a tour, there is no way to point out dangerous features. I had a coffee table made from a tree slab with pointed edges. I told them it was a wedding present, designed and hand crafted by my brother, and I was not going to get rid of it. They laughed, and I explained I had received many bruises by banging into it before I had a stroke.

As I did not have handles in our shower, they suggested I take a shower in the hospital the next morning without holding on to any hand rails. I did so, and passed! During their visit, they suggested I make oatmeal in our kitchen. I suggested I make tea, because I was tired of hospital tea made with water that was not at the boiling point. I used an electric tea kettle. This device fascinated them, and they enjoyed my tea. They approved of the rest of the house and thought I could easily walk down the four steps to the pool. They advised me to be very careful not to trip over our cats, who appeared glad to see me. This visit home was wonderful, and I appreciated the advice they gave me. Being a burro had led to an easy house to live in. The therapists drove me back to Boone Hospital Center, and I only had one

more night to stay there.
When I was discharged, I was ready to go home! I threw out the hospital flowers and packed! (I mention my flowers because a nurse said I remembered to do that, and I looked organized.) I was able to walk out the door of my room. I heard not many stroke victims could do that. I was asked the inevitable question about what was the first thing I was going to do when I went home. Ken had already made appointments to get my hair cut and for electrolysis for my chin. I lamented, "I am going to get my hair cut and my beard removed." That got a chuckle from a male physical therapist.
Coming home after being in the hospital for five weeks was a wonderful experience. Although I probably did many things you will not do, I believe several of them will be familiar. One of them was enjoying how wonderful our bed felt. Also, compared to the hospital, it was quiet. Nobody came to my bed wanting to draw blood. A nurse did not come every morning to wake me and give

me medicine. Sorrento, one of our cats, jumped on our bed at 7 a.m. to wake me. I could watch the morning TV program I enjoyed without being disturbed. I can only describe this "feeling at home" as wonderful. I could make tea using the electric tea kettle and go back to bed. In the hospital, breakfast was served at 7 a.m. I did not have to eat from a tray and hear the banging of cups, saucers, and plates. It was so quiet! From this wonderful morning, I progressed to enjoy our home. I did not know the extent of the hard details that were ahead.

I sure appreciated the home we had built. I enjoyed the beautiful scenery around our home. Little did I realize that making and pouring all the concrete during the building process would enable me to have a comfortable home environment. I was certainly thankful I had done all that hard work when I was able. As we had designed our home for retirement life, I knew, physically, life would be as easy as possible.

I was not aware about all the mental adjustments

I would have to make. I could not have survived without thinking about all the advice therapists, nurses, and physicians had given me. I really feel sorry for people who have a stroke and do not go to a rehabilitation unit. As I have said, everyone told me all strokes are different, but there are certain things almost everybody has to re-learn. I could dress myself at home, but Ken had to fasten my bra for months. Why did people invent bras? I did not require a walker and, at first, I tended to stay indoors. My concentration was poor, and I had trouble paying attention to details.

Cooking Again

My attention span and math skills were so poor Ken that did all our cooking. When I tried to cook, Ken was in the kitchen with me. Ken was afraid to leave me alone, which was totally justified because I was a disaster. Being in my own kitchen, which I had personally designed, was much more enjoyable than the hospital kitchen, but I certainly did not know how to cook or serve food. I could go on and on with these silly details, but they did make me feel totally incompetent. I had been cooking since I was ten years old, and Having a Ph.D. in food science, but these facts did not help me. I just had to be patient and keep practicing.

I felt the effects of my stroke had been cruel to me. Looking back, I guess I would have been in even more trouble if I had not learned to cook in the first place. The argument can then be made that learning something totally new would have been easier than re-learning everything. What I can say is I did want to cook without making mistakes. I burned some cheese bread under the broiler. I left a paper towel too close to the electric element and it almost burned. I turned on the wrong elements and forgot to turn them off. I tried to whip egg whites. They did not whip because I still had some egg yolk in the bowl. I could not figure out how to calculate 2/3 cup of butter. If I had a recipe that required four items, I would put in three items. I forgot to put the rum in the rum sauce.

Changing recipes was impossible for me to do. Therefore, I wanted to make the recipe without calculating any changes. I had trouble doubling the recipe. I could not even think about making 2/3 of a recipe. I had almost never use processed foods with instructions on the package, so that was not an option I wanted to use. If you enjoy processed foods, I certainly recommend using them. Since I have left the hospital, I have studied the packaging on processed foods. Many have clear instructions. They may be an option if your cooking skills are lacking. This can also be a choice if your spouse or partner does not know how to cook.

I was fortunate because Ken is an excellent cook. He could help me with calculations. We had a "game" in the kitchen when Ken would say, "If we made 3/4 of this recipe, how much milk would we need?" Sometimes I got the correct answer. When I cooked several things at once, I had difficulty getting food to the table when it was hot. Ken had to instruct me about how to set the oven and the timer. I had great difficulty getting the right number of plates, knives, and forks to the table. Remembering to take frozen food out of the freezer beforehand was impossible.

I am a food scientist with a hobby of entertaining! We did not have our traditional Canada Day—Independence Day party because I did not want to be in large crowds. I just thought I would be uncomfortable around many people. It took five months before I was prepared to try to entertain. I started with two friends. I wanted to do everything perfectly! So, I started with wine and cheese. Counting out four plates, cutlery, and having sufficient cheese was a challenge for me. Of course, I made some mistakes. Ken also noted I was not being a good hostess, being very uncomfortable assisting our guests. Afterwards, one of them commented I was making good use of my left hand and arm. The next time I entertained, I also had two friends, and I cooked menu items I was familiar with. Counting was again hard! Everything was served hot and in order. When Ken and I ate alone, I frequently forgot cutlery and counted the plates wrong. I am just talking about two people.

The next time I entertained, I tried four friends, and I had a disaster. I planned several menu items I had not previously prepared. I was hopeless about planning in what order to prepare the items. I had the table set for six, and Ken found me in the kitchen in turmoil. He told me to go and lie down, and he prepared several of the items. Our guests arrived, the food was served, and we had wonderful conversation. When they left, I said, "I am not going to have to count to six again!" Ken made an appropriate comment that not many people cook for six people anyway.

From then on, when I got confused in the kitchen, I just swore to relieve my frustration, and I slowly carried on. My abilities in the kitchen have slowly improved. In January 2004, I had to ask Ken how to cut grapefruit. When I learn how to do something, I remember it. So, one piece of advice is only entertain friends who know you are recovering from a stroke! I could not have entertained without Ken's assistance.

I am sure some people might wonder why I mention entertaining in this chapter. I did not need to entertain to help my recovery from a stroke. We had built our home with a large kitchen. Ken has a 20-gallon electric mixer for bread baking. We have a large dining room and living room that are comfortable for many friends. Outside of our home, we have attached patios where entertaining is easy on pleasant days. With the physical location of our home, and our enjoyment of being surrounded by friends and family, it was mentally important for me to entertain. When I could be successful, I felt psychologically better. When I had failures, I was determined I would do better the next time.

Making Some Expensive Mistakes

I made two very expensive disasters that were caused by my lack of having a good attention span. One of them anyone can do in their kitchen; the other serious one was in the vegetable garden.

A Flood in the Garden: Ken has a large vegetable garden that is located in a field away from our home. He has an irrigation system. One night, he asked me to go up to the garden and turn off the irrigation system. I said I would. Three days later, I went up to the garden to retrieve some tomatoes. Ken was just sitting there in the middle of his garden on a bucket. A flood surrounded him. Making matters worse, the power had gone out that day. The power truck had driven through the flood to reach the power lines. So, later Ken had to get his tractor and fill up the ruts left by the truck tires. I had run 30,000 gallons of water. The water company eventually sent us a letter to inquire if perhaps we had a leak because our bill was so large.

Cleaning the Refrigerator: At 4 p.m. one day, I turned off the refrigerator because I was going to clean it. The next morning, Ken found water all over the kitchen. This was the day after he had discovered his flood. I heard him lament, "Now what do I have to fix?" Thankfully, he only had to replenish the ice machine, and our food was not destroyed.

Outdoor Challenges

There are so many things I had done for years, that now I could not figure out how to do. Outdoors was a challenge. I am sure some of you would think, "Why should I worry about being outdoors?" As I mentioned when I recovered after my heart surgery, I love the location where we built our home. I like gardening. I enjoy the trees when they are blooming. I tolerate weeding because there is no other option. Being outdoors gives me a refreshed feeling. I do not like it when bugs bite me, but I also have to tolerate them. I have very sensitive skin, so I always wear sunscreen and a cap with a visor, as well as lotion to prevent chigger and tick bites. When spring arrives, I am usually outside as much as possible. I did not want having a stroke to deprive me of our garden. However, many challenges confronted me. I could not figure out how to tie up Ken's tomato plants that grow to be about five feet high. I have tied them up for 30 years, but I could not do it. Ken got so frustrated that he had to physically show me how. When I received instructions, sometimes patiently, I could accomplish them.

I had trouble starting the lawn mower. Ken watched me and was amused when I got to a corner and had difficulty figuring out which direction to turn. Since I have had open-heart surgery, I have not yet tried to use a weed eater. I believe the vibration would hurt my chest. Now that I am on Coumadin, I most certainly will not try the weed eater.

I had trouble being thorough when I was weeding. I could use the weed probe with my left hand. Sitting on my knees was uncomfortable. Each summer, I have to be patient enough to remove all the weeds. When we bought a few new trees, Ken had to dig the holes. During the hot summer months, I could not carry buckets of water to our special trees because they were too heavy to lift.

I could not put the garden hoses in the correct spots. I got mixed up with the ends. All of these things I had easily done correctly before! My days of being a burro are past!

Because we built our home, I do not want to purchase a condo or apartment and avoid these outdoor challenges. Going out in our small boat on the lake was another challenge. I do not have a good sense of balance on the boat. I am also afraid to drive the boat. For safety's sake, I should learn how to drive it. When we went on boating trips during the summer, Ken did all the work. When Ken tried to get me to drive, I opposed him, saying I had learned to drive a car that summer and that was enough. During the fall, when the leaves were at their peak color, Ken and I took a boat ride on a warm day. As my abilities in the boat are limited, I packed the sandwiches and enjoyed the day with him. Being in good company is also important!

Swimming Again

With all the activities I could not do, I had to swim

again. This time, I had limited strength in my left side, and I could not swim in a straight line. The exercises I received from the physical therapist helped me. I was really terrified to go into the water until I went with a physical therapist. However, now I never swim without a lifeguard! I knew that all along. I learned that as a Girl Guide years ago, but it is just one of those things to which I did not pay attention. Several of my friends who are master swimmers assisted me. I need a lot of improvement, but I continue to splash away! I think when I swim. I wrote much of this book while I was swimming.

Hiking With Friends

One of my friends who visited me in the inpatient rehabilitation ward had said, "See you on the trail." At that point, I did not even know if I would be able to walk out of the hospital room. When I could eventually go to the trail in our town for our traditional hike on Monday mornings, everyone realized we should change our term hiking to walking. They walked slowly with me. They showed me they were concerned about me, and they knew I had returned as soon as I could! My friends changed their pace so I could keep up with them. We found benches to sit on and had coffee breaks after our exercise. Being with my friends on Monday mornings was important to me because it meant I was slowly returning to normal. As I could not yet drive, they kindly took turns driving me to our trail. The feeling of normalcy was important to me. I was physically okay to walk, but the fact that I was able to walk with friends was gratifying.

Your Enlightenment

Enjoy doing things in your home and outdoors that you are physically and mentally able to do and used to enjoy. You could make some expensive mistakes. Be patient with yourself, and realize you will make errors. Swear, if that makes you feel better. A great deal of satisfaction comes from doing things in a manner that pleases you. Be as physically active as you are able to be. Consult with your physical therapists. I started to hike and swim before I was ready, but I enjoy being challenged, and I did not do any physical harm to myself. Take an initial effort as soon as you are ready. Do not wait until you are completely recovered before trying a task. Your mental state will be helped by your efforts. You will have a better sense of your well-being.

5

Five: Having a Supportive Spouse

I can only start this chapter by emphasizing that, after you have a stroke, you need a spouse or partner to assist you 24/7. I am so fortunate that Ken is available for me. Of course, I felt hurt when I thought he was not patient enough. On the other hand, I thought that Ken was too protective. I have these feelings because I have always lived a very independent life, except when I had heart surgery. When I began to observe Ken's actions while I was in the hospital, I realized that my health had affected him for a second time. His life was totally changed. I would sometimes think "in sickness and in health." A former Ph.D. student called me from Sudan and reassured me that I had helped Ken when I was a burro; now it was his turn. I realized what she meant, but Ken did not need any motivation to give me assistance.

When I told my brother, Frank, that I was thinking about writing this book, he said, "the title is simple: *Marry Ken*."

I acknowledged Ken's help in the acknowledgements to this book. His help has made my life enjoyable. You can use this chapter to make "lists" when your partner or spouse asks what they can do to be of assistance.

Ken's Actions in the Hospital

Ken answered all my questions. When I came out of shock, I wanted to know everything. Ken told me that I had not been able to sign my name when he took me to the emergency room. He told me that I said I was freezing when they moved me into the CT scan. He said that I could not put my left finger to my nose. He did not see me take an EEG. He explained that I would not stay in bed and I fainted with three nurses in the bathroom.

Apparently, I asked him the same questions many, many times, for it was important for me to understand. I could not understand the first time he answered my questions so I asked them again. When he told me something foolish that I had done, I wanted to know if I had really done it. Ken went with me to the rehabilitation unit and helped answer questions about my health and medications. Ken communicated with our family and friends, and they started to visit.

Ken brought my clothes to the hospital. As I was used to wearing suits and lab coats, I wanted to dress in coordinated clothes. Actually, I did not like the fact that Ken would have to hunt through my cupboards and drawers to find everything. They should have been organized, and they were not!

As I did not have any diet restrictions, Ken brought food on many occasions. Nurses would usually say, "Your pizza smells so good." Getting relief from hospital food was great! Initially, the nurses told Ken that they were afraid I had forgotten how to eat as I was not eating hospital food. So, Ken brought in a half-pound of peeled shrimp, which we consumed for dinner, and the staff was no longer afraid that I had forgotten how to eat. Ken's frequent visits were very important, and I wanted to know when he would return. I looked forward to hearing gossip. He explained to our friends that they should not telephone because I was lifting the telephone upside down.

Ken took my laundry home. When I had the myxoma removed, Ken did not know how to wash clothes. I used to make a joke that he had repaired the washing machine, but had never used it. This time, instructions were not necessary.

Ken shared tales about our three Russian Blue cats, Sorrento, Comox and Tofino. I sure missed them! Since my heart surgery, Sointula had died, and we adopted two new kittens, Tofino and Comox. I named our cats after towns in British Columbia. I have friends who visit these towns when they go to British Columbia. I told our veterinarian I was going to mention our cats in this book, and he said, "Great, Hemingway did!" I wish I could write as well as Hemingway. I would rather have had Sorrento climb up onto my bed to wake me each morning instead of the nurse in the inpatient rehabilitation unit. I guess I frequently told her that.

As I had recently retired, I wanted to know the latest campus developments. Ken cancelled my appointments, including my retirement party, and went in my place to handle some of my meetings including the Scandinavian Heritage Society.

Ken shared current events with me. Operation Iraqi Freedom started while I was in the rehabilitation unit, so we had much to discuss as events unfolded. I became consumed with Operation Iraqi Freedom. When I was alone, my TV was on constantly. We were expecting so many disasters. Would the weapons of mass destruction be biological or would they be chemical or nuclear?

Would our troops be safe? It is amazing that the weapons of mass destruction were never found. First thing in the morning, I wanted to learn about the night's developments. I was mesmerized by these events. If I had been home, I would probably just have had time to watch the highlights. My neurologist knew that I was constantly watching Operation Iraqi Freedom coverage. He interviewed me about "today's developments." Really, he was conducting a neurological assessment to determine how I was doing. I passed!

Ken's days were largely consumed by the activities he did for me. He continued to do some metal work, but all of his other projects were postponed. Having recently retired, he had planned many projects to accomplish in the spring. Of course, he had previously expected that I would help him with many of these projects. I constantly heard him on the phone saying, "Nan is going to be okay." Little did he know at that point that I would eventually recover! I knew that Ken was having a difficult time worrying. He is one of those lucky people that lose weight when they worry. By the time he took me home from Boone Hospital Center, he had lost ten pounds.

I dreaded that Ken would find out how poorly I was doing in my therapy sessions. As professors, we had similar careers. We both taught and did research. We were active in service projects with our university. I used to be able to keep up with him. Now I felt foolish and dreaded his visits to observe how I was doing with the therapists. They explained how Ken should help at home. I knew that he needed to know, but I did not want to appear such a failure. I even had a dream that he needed a psychiatrist to learn how to deal with such a different wife. The therapists always told him that I was making good progress. Ken had to witness the progression from the time when he found me in my confused state, the transition from a wheelchair with "George," to a wheelchair without "George," to a walker, and to walking with support from a therapist. He saw me when I could not read and when I could. He observed many of my emotional swings, from total devastation to being positive about our future. Ken had a hard role to play, without the knowledge that I would continue to improve. I was aware that Ken's life had been changed. I personally resolved to not be more dependent than necessary.

One week before my discharge, Ken was asked to spend a week participating in my therapy sessions as part of a special program the inpatient rehabilitation unit. During physical therapy, he listened closely to their instructions. During recreational therapy, we had to play a word puzzle. He excelled, and I struggled. During speech therapy, I was given an assignment that included recording grades in a book. Although there were only six names, I could not do it. Luckily, I had retired, or I would have given grades of A to all of my 130 students! Therapists helped me in the rehabilitation unit, but my home life was a mystery to them. They did not know if I would retain everything they had taught me. Many of their instructions implied I should always remember their guidance.

Ken Facilitates My Life At Home

As you can tell, I had been a very independent person, so it was hard to accept that I needed constant attention. Ken would not leave me alone in the house in case I had an accident, like fall in the shower, have trouble getting out of the whirlpool bath, forget to turn off my hair curler, and everything else he could think of that I might do by mistake. I spent most of the time in the house because I was afraid of falling outdoors while my balance steadily improved.

Ken cooked all our meals. When I began to help, I had some disasters, which I have explained previously. Ken drove me to the grocery store. Having Ken shop with me was one of my most unpleasant experiences. I like to shop with a vague list. As an engineer, Ken likes to shop with a complete list. I buy whatever I want. Ken always checks the prices. I have the "fun" approach. So, during our frequent visits, I had to follow his approach. I had to hold the cart and stand beside him while he made the selection. A few times, I would wander off. He told me I was acting like a little child, getting lost.

I found the meaning of prices hard to comprehend. I could not take $1.40 and multiply it by five! Enough said about this unpleasantness! I look upon it as a nightmare. When I got my driver's license again, the first thing I wanted to do was go to the grocery store without Ken!

Ken drove me to my appointments and to outpatient therapy, and waited patiently, reading many books. I usually enjoyed driving myself, so having Ken drive me everywhere was a degrading experience. I hated that I had lost my independence. My freedom was gone! Ken goes on organized trips, keeping everything in a logical order. He even insisted that I number our stops, which was confusing.

Ken kept track of our calendar. I made some mistakes putting appointments on the incorrect day. I always liked to be punctual, so receiving calls that I had missed an appointment was frustrating. Ken double-checked all my appointments.

Ken checked my outgoing mail. When I came home, I could not put the stamp, address and return address on each envelope. My friends said I sent them the correct "thank you" notes, but it was a huge task. I had trouble putting the correct size card in the right envelope. I thought I could do this trivial job myself, but one card came back to me because I had forgotten to stamp it. So, Ken always checked before I mailed a letter.

Ken oversaw that I took the correct medicine, which I frequently forgot to take. I also got days confused. I was prescribed Coumadin, a blood thinner that is very difficult to control. It is crucial that I remember to take it at 4 p.m. every day. Many things affect it, such as foods that contain vitamin K, which I now have to avoid.

We purchased a weekly pill organizer, which had the day of the week and the time for taking the medicine. As I continued to make mistakes, Ken made me a form for each week where I could write an "x" when I had taken the right pills at the right time. I also bought a watch that had the day of the week on it as well as the date. Having such a device is crucial! So, the form Ken made me and the pill organizer gave both of us two checks for errors.

Initially, Ken filled my pill organizer. I was not even capable of doing that! During the last week on the rehabilitation unit, I was given a list of my medications and was instructed to ask for them. Unfortunately, that learning did not transfer to my life at home.

When I came home, Ken had to do the unpleasant task of replacing our cat litter because it was too heavy for me to dump. This had always been my task and Ken hated doing it! I resumed this task as soon as I was able. I only mention this because, when you have something too heavy for you to do, get help with it!

Fortunately, we have a person who cleans our house, so it was in great shape when I returned. It took me six months before I felt I could dust the china and not break anything. Ken cleaned the heavy crystal so I would not drop it. I remember him asking, "How many more pieces of crystal do I have to wash?" My answer was "24" and he continued.

When the house cleaner forgot to clean a toilet, I started to clean it. I could not remember how! I slowly figured it out. The neat thing is that once I learned how to do something, I remembered how from then on. One time I had to ask our cleaner how to wash the kitchen floor, as I had totally forgotten.

When I arrived home, we had a new system for getting into our e-mail account. It took me six months before my attention span was good enough to use the new system.

Ken planted our spring flowers in pots. I enjoy planting my spring flowers by "muddling." Ken uses the "engineering" approach where it is done efficiently. When Ken planted our flowers, I was constantly thinking about the pansies I was directed to plant when I was in the rehabilitation unit. I could have physically planted my own flowers in pots once I had made all the difficult choice decisions, but it would have taken me hours. Ken's help in the nursery and his efficiency were appreciated. The plants looked great and lasted in the patio pots until fall, but in future years I planned on doing it independently, with the "muddling" approach.

Ken mowed our grass because I was too inefficient. I tried to weed, but my attention span was not sufficient to do a thorough job, so Ken spent hours thoroughly weeding. Previously, I explained how hard it was to concentrate on weeding. We had planted some buffalo grass that had to be thoroughly weeded for the first two years after it was planted, so this task was crucial. There are many things we would not have planted if we had known I would have a stroke. I guess I can use that scenario with numerous things.

Fortunately, Ken will not shop for clothes with me. A dear friend took me clothes shopping when I could not drive. She did not know that I had trouble getting my left arm into sweaters or jackets. We went to a nearby store and I started to try on some clothes. When my friend realized what trouble I was having and came in to help, laughter and giggles came out of the dressing room. We told the sales person about my troubles. She was most understanding and told us to take as long as we needed. Whenever I return to that store, she remembers!

Living at home is much different now. I hate thinking slowly. My memory is not impaired, but thinking at a snail's pace is very difficult. I do my best to be congenial, but sometimes I just lose my cool and cannot contain my temper. I understand why Ken gets frustrated with me, but it is hard to state things clearly. Ken will say, "Don't you even understand that?" One day, Ken asked me for an egg. I said, "Do you want a whole one?" Ken replied that one-half of an egg would do. Why do I say such foolish things?

For example, in November 2003, several of us were packaging some venison. I told everyone that they should date the meat 1993, but it was late 2003! While we were packing the meat,

I got a phone call from a friend who normally comes to swim with me. I told him to come out, even though we were having a storm with lightning and thunder. I had forgotten the impact of lightning.

I said, "How can I be so foolish, and think so slowly?" Ken said, "That is why we are all here to keep you straight."

Your Enlightenment

Many friends have told me their husbands would not be as good at taking care of them as Ken continues to be with me. This was the second time Ken had to take extra care of me. I believe my father would be pleased with what Ken has done for me. When you have a stroke, it happens while you are living your life. In my case, Ken has been wonderful. It took him a concerted nine months to help me with my "recovery," and I am still making many improvements. He will not travel without me. I would like to tell him that he is being overprotective. But, if I did that, I would make a foolish mistake.

If you do not have a supportive spouse to help you, you will need a good friend or partner.

Perhaps you can list all the activities that Ken did for me if they ask, "What can I do to help?"

I had no idea it would take so much effort to recover from a stroke. Without Ken's support, I would not have the quality of life I am enjoying today.

Ken and I continue to have a very strong relationship. We usually enjoy doing the same things. Ken has to help me more than he ever did before. I wish that were not so, but I have to accept help on a continual basis. My personal goal is to never be more dependent than I just have to be and stay as physically strong as I am capable of being.

6

Six: Outpatient Therapy to Help Myself

When I was discharged from Boone Hospital Center, it was recommended that I continue with physical, occupational and speech therapies. My health insurance company approved 60 sessions with a co-pay for the next year. That meant I had 20 sessions with each therapist if needed.

When I began outpatient sessions, I was re-assessed to determine my current condition for each different therapy. My speech therapist was the only therapist I worked with after discharge who had treated me on the rehabilitation unit, so she knew the extent of my struggles. I was thrilled that she had been assigned to me.

Special Advice from Outpatient Therapists

In June 2003, I had an appointment with the speech therapist and I told her that I was excited that the feeling was coming back on my left side. She asked what my symptoms were, and I said I was tingling from head to toe on the left side. She told me that it was a symptom of another stroke and rushed me to the emergency ward. Ken was outside the Boone Hospital Center patiently waiting for the end of my visit. An EEG was immediately ordered. I had the hospital technician find Ken, as that test would take at least an hour. I can imagine how terrified he was. An Electroencephalography (EEG) is a simple, painless procedure in which 20 wires (leads) are pasted on the scalp to trace and record the brain's electrical activity. Recordings in the form of wave patterns also help identify epilepsy and certain rare metabolic brain diseases.

When I came into the room to have the EEG done, the technician burst into laughter when she saw me. Of course, I was wondering why. She said that she had worked with me on February 27, 2003 and I had been the worst patient she had ever had. Apparently, when she put the electrodes on my head, I tore them off. When she told me to keep still so that the test would work, I constantly moved around. This time I followed her instructions.

The neurologist also ordered an MRI of my brain as soon as it could be done. So, I had to wait another week to see if I had had another stroke. An MRI is an extremely difficult test, as it requires lying very still in a closed space. I hear that patients are frequently medicated so it will be easier.

To give a definition, magnetic resonance imaging (MRI) of the brain is performed by placing a patient's head in a confined space and generating a very powerful magnetic field that produces exquisitely detailed anatomic images. No x-rays are involved and the MRI is extremely safe. MRI is better than CT (computed tomography, another kind of imaging technology) for detecting certain serious problems, such as previous strokes.

Sometimes a contrast agent (a substance that shows clearly on an MRI image) is injected into a patient's veins to further enhance the images. No contrast agent was used for my MRI.

Computer models are used to measure how the brain functions. The major disadvantages of MRI are its expense and the time required. MRI cannot be used by patients who are claustrophobic. During my test, I had a small window to look out if I chose. I had to hear clanging and banging as the magnets surrounded me. A technician was always there talking to me, telling me how much longer the test would take. I appreciated her voice.

The computer results were sent to my neurologist, where I was soon scheduled for a visit. He told me no new strokes had been found, and I was instructed to continue with my outpatient therapy.

Speech Therapy

I met with my speech pathologist two days per week. For the weekend, she gave me extensive homework. The main comment she made to me was, compared to how I had been on the rehabilitation unit, she could see that this time I really wanted to learn and always tried to pay attention.

We continued with math up until the sixth grade level. At home, I took hours doing homework assignments. Long division was the hardest math task, and I spent hours doing it. This time I was back in my home office with cats to stroke when I needed to try to reduce my frustration level. Again, I was graded by my speech therapist. On the average, I got about fifty percent. I also did more complex word problems than I had done on the rehab unit, which I enjoyed much more than rigorous math exercises. When I correctly solved problems, it gave me more confidence that I would be able to handle situations as they arose in my life, which I needed. Regaining my ability to work with numbers was a tremendous effort.

I can honestly say that I worked as hard as I could to improve myself. I did not play hooky with my homework, and I was very diligent. Of course, I made mistakes with math but I genuinely tried to improve. In her office, the speech therapist started to time me to sharpen my skills. Being timed caused a great deal of pressure and I made more mistakes.

I did many things in her office that were not directly related to math. One day she said, "How are you with the telephone book?" I said, "Terrible. How did you know that would be a problem?"

She grinned, and we began to read the telephone book together. I also had to read airplane and bus schedules. I told her that reading the TV schedule and lining up the programs with the times was frustrating. I had spent my academic life doing statistical tables where the columns and lines are matched. I was not even going to think about doing statistics, but I had to learn how to correctly match columns with lines. One revelation came when I could really understand the reason for carrying numbers when I was doing math.

She gave me two standardized tests to determine

cognitive ability. I was extremely nervous for both of these tests. I thought about having my Ph.D. exam, when I thought that was the last examination I was ever going to have. For both of these exams, spaced three weeks apart, my cognitive abilities were judged. I was borderline normal. Being told that I was assessed as borderline normal was a hard fact to take. As the two tests were standardized, I had to believe the results. The results hurt, and they still do. I have functioned well throughout my life, and now I know that I will not be able to live as I have been accustomed to.

My insurance company would not pay for any more sessions of speech therapy, as I was considered "functional." That was not how I felt, so my therapist recommended some books to buy and use at home. I bought them, and went to a school store to purchase some word problem books. I was clearly at the sixth grade level, which I remember telling a friend on the phone. He was familiar with my academic career, during which I had published numerous papers using statistics. He asked me, "Is sixth grade good?" I assured him that it certainly was, as I had come from first grade to the sixth grade within five months.

I greatly benefited from having the same speech therapist. For the next four months, I got up early in the morning to do math. I stopped my early morning math practice when I decided to write this book. I purchased some computer programs for mastering problem-solving skills and building math confidence at the 6th grade level. I also need to learn how to do crossword puzzles.

Physical Therapy

When the first physical therapist assessed me, she observed how I walked and determined my balance by having me stand on my toes. She gave me exercises for "my trunk" that I could do at home. Together, we made the decision that my limited number of therapy sessions should be allocated to speech and occupational therapy, where I could later learn to drive. I requested aqua-therapy exercises as I knew I was afraid to swim. Each morning, Ken drove me to the pool and observed patients waddling into the building on a ramp with side rails. The physical therapist who taught me specializes in aqua-exercises and is there on a daily basis. He walked me around the shallow end and directed me to perform certain exercises. I could do them immediately.

The therapist gave me two one-hour sessions in the pool. First, I was directed to do exercises that would help my sense of balance and strengthen my left leg and arm. I did all these exercises using both sides of my body. He told me that dual exercises are always recommended so that I would gain uniform strength on each side of my body. He gave me diagrams of these exercises so I could perform them in our pool at home.

He also swam with me at the deep end of the pool. As he was beside me, I was excited I could actually swim. He told me I was a good swimmer and assured me I would have no problems, provided I always had a lifeguard. Putting my head in the water and swimming was a wonderful experience. I could not have done it without the presence of a physical therapist.

Swimming with a Crooked Style

I was instructed to alternate the exercises I was taught by the therapist with swimming, which would be difficult at first. Once I began them at home, I had oodles of energy. Ken made some large wooden paddles to use in the water to help strengthen my arms. Basically, all the exercises caused my body to move, keeping my head out of the water. When I was being a burro, and dreaming about having a pool, I had no idea I would use it to recover from open-heart surgery, and then a stroke.

I spent my time in the pool mastering the prescribed exercises, as well as swimming, almost every day, with Ken as my lifeguard. I had to be considerate of Ken's time, as watching me for 20 minutes was a boring activity. I had trouble swimming because my left side was not strong enough.

Thus, I swam crooked. I have a friend who is a master swimmer who comes to swim with me on a regular basis. I continue to improve! When you swim crooked, you cannot easily swim half a mile and burn up all the calories I always need to. No matter my style, swimming is always my favorite exercise!

Walking With Enthusiasm

My physical therapist told me I could walk with friends. If I went too far and eventually limped on my left side, I was instructed to take a rest and not walk so far the next time. My kind friends walked slowly, as everyone was very concerned. At last I could walk with my friends! Many of us have been "hiking" every Monday, whether it is hot, cold, dry or rainy. I was doing something enjoyable! That was much better than lying in a hospital bed thinking about hiking. When I could not drive, they picked me up at home every Monday morning and drove me to the trail across town. Being on our trail, smelling and seeing nature, exercising and catching up on news was great!

Occupational Therapy

As I could dress myself and had help living at home, I wanted to concentrate on learning to drive for the second time. In the state of Missouri, my driver's license was not taken from me, but I was told by a social worker that I should not drive. Six months after my stroke, my neurologist scheduled me for a driving assessment, which I requested. I've been told that neurologists wait until patients make this request before they authorize the occupational therapists to assist them. I believe this procedure assures the neurologists they are mentally ready for the challenge of driving.

My Driving Assessment

Before I left the rehabilitation unit, a nurse told me not to rush and to be sure I was ready to drive again. I did not like her advice because being driven and losing my independent lifestyle was very difficult for me. When my good Canadian friends visited me in June 2003, I also told them I was going to learn to drive the next week. They told me it was too early so I waited, again. One of them is an occupational and physical therapist, so I knew I had to respect her opinion. When Ken drove with me down our long driveway, my reaction times were too slow, I did not know what the park function was, and I stayed away from the road. Finally, in August 2003, I told my neurologist I was ready!

Before I took the test, I had to have my eyes examined. There had been a lot of changes in them since my stroke, and new glasses were prescribed. During my driving assessment, I had many assignments. First, I was asked to copy a diagram of a house. I forgot to copy the windows. Second, I was asked to explain driving signs. I could do this, but I had trouble with the one that said, "Yield on Green." I had to remember I would use this at a green light. Third, I was given a test where

I had to draw similar lines together, where each line had to be equal length. Fourth, I was given a test to determine whether I could do two things simultaneously. I had to integrate numbers and letters, which was hard. I was told that I had to mix numbers and letters in a logical pairing up to 59. I got as far as 1A, 2B, 3C, 4D, 5E, 6F, 7G. I was totally confused. There was no way I could have gone as far as 59! All of these tests were timed, which increased my personal levels of pressure.

My reflex tests were next. I stood in a dark room and lights came on a large board. The lights came from all directions – top, bottom, left, and right. They came on at different speeds that were determined by the occupational therapist. My assignment was to use my fists and turn out the lights as soon as I saw them. I thought this was a very sensible test, as having fast reflexes is crucial to good driving. The summary score of my driving assessment was 201. I had to score 200 points before I was eligible to have an on-road test with an instructor, which we scheduled for two days later.

As I had a valid driver's license, Ken took me on several back roads to help get ready for the driving test. I knew he wanted me to pass this test, as driving me everywhere from February 26 to August 14, 2003 had been a long burden for him.

I mastered the car okay on the roads, but I was occasionally too close to the sides of other cars. I drove too fast, as I normally did. The night before my test, I was very worried. Getting a score of 201 did not increase my level of confidence. Ken told me I should do everything I could to have loads of concentration during the road test the next day.

On the day of the test, the driving instructor could not have been nicer. He had a car with an emergency brake in case he needed it. He assessed the strength of my left side. We started out in a parking lot where I familiarized myself with the car. The occupational therapist sat in the back seat. We drove around the city, including the highway, and a large parking lot for about one hour. All the time, the therapist and the driving instructor were chatting. Afterwards, they told me they thought I would fail the on-road driving test because I could not do two things at once, i.e., integrating numbers and letters. They gave me clear directions about where to turn throughout our town and on the highway.

The driving instructor soon said that I was a "Type A" driver, I enjoyed driving, and I had trouble telling left and right. In that short time, he had figured out my driving habits. That gave me confidence in his skills.

When we returned to Boone Hospital Center, both the therapist and instructor signed a form that I had passed. That record will now be kept with the neurologist in case I ever need it for a liability case. Having a reconstructed heart and a stroke would not make an accident easy to explain unless I had official authorization to drive.

The instructor and occupational therapist gave me some good instructions. I was to be careful that I did not leave a stop sign too fast, and, of course, I was not supposed to go beyond the speed limit. I had passed my test and I no longer had to rely on Ken and my friends to drive me! The therapists told me to drive short distances at first and rest when I got home. When driving, you are doing many things at the same time. Over time, driving becomes automatic and you forget how many senses are involved.

Wonderful Exhaustion!

I was totally exhausted after my driver's test! Of all of the tests/exams I have had since my stroke, this test made me feel the best. Ken drove me to lunch afterward. When we got home, I went into the dining room and put my head on the table in total exhaustion. The date was August 14, 2003. You may remember this day, as the power system on the eastern side of Canada and the U.S. was lost. I saw all the trouble on TV and thought "terrorists" until I heard the real news.

Ken gave me some sensible advice about driving. At first, he drove with me for short trips. I came home exhausted every time. My brother came from Calgary and drove with me in the dark. That was a disconcerting sensation. We came home through winding country roads.

When I took the car out alone, I did not remember how to get gasoline. It took me six trips to figure out how to use my credit card to pay at the pump. After my first stop for gasoline, I neglected to put the gas cap on, and had to purchase another cap. When I was first able to drive myself to meet my hiking friends, they realized how worried I was. They treated me to coffee and a huge muffin after our hike. When I drove home after the large muffin, I sat at an intersection with my heart racing, trying to decide where to turn. A friend called that afternoon to make sure I had made it home. Since then, I have not had the same fear. I laugh whenever I go through this intersection.

When I drove my uncle during his visit to our city, I told him to be quiet as I did not want to have any distractions. He hated how cautious I was.

Alone Again: What a Sense of Freedom!

I could finally drive alone, as long as I told Ken where I was going. He needed assurance that I would be okay.

Taking the drivers assessment exam was extremely valuable to me. Without the direction and advice of the occupational therapists and the driving instructor, I would not have the level of confidence that I needed to drive well. I do not have any driving restrictions. However, I have made two for myself. First, I am not going to drive on the interstate system. Even before I had a stroke, I was becoming afraid. Second, I am not going to drive with any children as passengers. I feel very fortunate that I did not hurt anyone when I had a stroke. It could have happened when I was driving.

With my success, I had such an elated feeling. It reminded me of when I had defended my Ph.D. examination. Deserved success is a priceless feeling.

Your Enlightenment

For me, the term "outpatient" means to continue to do as much as you are physically and mentally capable of doing. If you have the same therapist you had in the hospital, that might be of benefit. Take all the advice competent therapists and physicians give, for they have helped thousands of people recover and have prescribed corrective methods for you. The professionals have studied intensively for this purpose. The procedures that were recommended for me may be quite different for you.

I drove them crazy with questions. I even asked if studying math would help with other areas in my brain. When the therapist said, "Yes!", It gave me a positive feeling. Many times I have thought it would be better to sit cuddling a cat instead of exercising or doing math problems, but my conscience will not let me! So, exercise first and then do something else that will reduce your stress levels. Of all the advice I have given, do things that please you most and will reduce your levels of stress. Not one of the therapists or physicians gave me any advice that seemed ridiculous throughout my outpatient therapy sessions. Always ask what their purpose is in giving an exercise/ test. When they explain their reasons for a testing process, try to realize why the standardized test is necessary for your progression. Unfortunately, I had to learn to accept some bad results. The stigma of being "borderline normal" will always be with me. Hopefully, your results will be better.

Whatever your health status or driving restrictions after a stroke, follow those restrictions to the best of your ability. Why risk hurting anyone?

During my academic life, I would have gone to

the library to verify what outpatient therapists told me. Now, I trust their professions, because their help has been superb.

Do every physical exercise you are capable of. Make sure you do not do anything that makes you sore. It is my opinion that you should not feel "perfectly strong" before you try to exercise, however a therapist may tell you the opposite, so listen to them. Consider your mental state, and how you can justify your sense of well-being.

Do not drive a car without passing your driver's assessment! You just have to put up with losing your independence as long as it takes. You will feel elated when you have the ability to drive again!

7

Seven: Enjoying a Driving Trip after a Stroke

I have referred to the term "genuine encouragement" frequently throughout this book. Receiving genuine encouragement is much more rewarding than just receiving encouragement. The concept became increasingly important to me throughout my journey, so I decided to share my comments about it in this chapter. Here is one of my personal equations:

GENUINE ENCOURAGEMENT = MOTIVATION TO RECOVER

Genuine encouragement can only be given by those who know you well. In my professional life, it happened when I gave a talk that spurred discussion with others about the topic. I have a fond memory of having a special professor who had been on my Ph.D. committee, thanking me and saying to my audience, "I hope you realize what she has been saying to you." To prepare for that lecture, and to come up with ideas, I had gone to the Rocky Mountains in Alberta and looked at the magnificent nature that surrounded me. Professionally, I received genuine encouragement from my colleagues whenever I published a paper with vital concepts in it.

After having a stroke, I first received genuine encouragement from my internal medicine physician as I was leaving the rehabilitation unit. I asked him if I was really doing well. His emphatic response was, "Yes, I have been with you every morning while you have been trying to put on your make-up for five weeks, and you are responding well to your situation." By that time, he knew me well enough to give me genuine encouragement and I accepted it as such.

I received genuine encouragement in June 2003

when two of my Canadian friends came to visit. I knew that their purpose was to personally assess me. The three of us celebrated our first birthdays together and have always felt close, despite the long distances we live from each other. Today, e-mail enables us to communicate with ease. During their delightful visit, they were pleased at the progress I was making. They cautioned me to observe the challenges that lay before me. As I have mentioned in the acknowledgements, they gave me the idea to write this book. They have since told me they knew writing was something I enjoyed doing and they wanted me to feel good about doing something that would help me improve. As I have written previously, I thought their suggestion was "nuts," as I had decided I was just going to find a way to enjoy my retirement. Their love and encouragement was genuine.

Staying With Relatives

In October 2003, Ken and I drove 600 miles to visit relatives. As we had decided, Ken did all the driving.

It was wonderful to have the opportunity to leave home. Being home was great, as by that time I had learned to function well, but we needed some new travel experiences. I was the "navigator." Once off the interstate, the numbers on the roads were confusing. We sometimes had one road with two numbers, and a junction point with letters. No wonder our foreign students have trouble driving on our roads. There was only one point where I was totally lost, and I could not tell Ken what direction to go.

When we were near our destination, I became very nervous. That did not make sense to me, as I know our relatives very well and enjoy spending time with them. As four of them are nurses, I did not want to appear a fool in front of them. Everyone appreciated all of the things Ken was doing to help me!

Our relatives gave me genuine encouragement. They knew me well enough to give me their honest opinions. Thus, I was relieved to receive such encouragement and advice. The emotion they demonstrated was important. Emotions sure make a difference. I told them that I felt compelled to write this book. They agreed it was necessary, as they had helped stroke patients who did not have enough details about what lay ahead of them. So on the drive home, I thought about details that I planned to share in this book.

They had several parties for us. I asked them appropriate questions and I remembered their answers. I remembered all their names and enjoyed talking to them. I felt very comfortable once my nervousness had disappeared. I told a teenager I was doing math at the sixth grade level. She just shook her head, trying to understand.

Ken's uncle and aunt drove us to a campus Ken's father had attended. Twenty-five years ago, he had received an honorary doctorate, so it was refreshing to be there again. It was nice to remember how proud he had been on the day he had received his honor. When we drove to that campus, I enjoyed sitting in the back seat and I did not have to navigate.

In our relative's homes, I frequently thought about the advice the therapists had given. I was extra cautious in showers. I was more tense, because we were always in a hurry. That was the first time that I realized pressure would really affect my ability to make decisions. When I was home, I had more time to think slowly. Ken's aunt took me shopping and I took way too long finding the "right" suit for a special occasion. Previously, I could make fast decisions. She was incredibly understanding as I persevered in buying a suit.

Ken and I left the city where our relatives lived and drove to see an exquisite home built by Frank Lloyd Wright, located in Pennsylvania. That first visit to *Falling Water* was important to us. The home we had built had many of the same features. Our home can be classified as organic architecture. If any of you have seen a picture of *Falling Water*, it was probably taken in the fall. We were there on a beautiful fall day. I will always remember the wonderful sound of the waterfall under the house. Ken really appreciated seeing the engineering detail drawings used for complete renovation of the home. I enjoyed all the features of the house. It is a neat feeling to finally see something you have always wanted to see.

Learning New Things in a Motel

During the visit to *Falling Water*, we stayed in a motel. That was the first motel or hotel I had been in since my stroke. I was going to rest for a bit, so Ken set the alarm clock and stepped out. When it went off, I thought it was a smoke detector! Ken was surprised when he returned in a very short time and found I had dressed and was getting ready to go out the door!

I had forgotten many things. I had to concentrate on finding our correct room number, and I had to learn how to put the plastic key card in the motel door. I had to learn where to put dollar bills in vending machines. Many times, I was just thinking about the advice I had received from therapists, and I was trying to pay attention and make fast decisions. Pressure hindered my ability to make decisions that were correct for us.

The ten day trip was very successful one, but ten days was long enough! I enjoyed coming home to our cats, Sorrento, Comox, and Tofino. They had been well cared for during our trip and were also very friendly when we returned.

Your Enlightenment

For your first driving trip, have someone else drive. As much as possible, do not drive in unfamiliar locations. Visit friends or family you know, who will plan some activities you enjoy. Try to remember what your therapists told you about living safely. Remember that you will be stressed in unfamiliar surroundings and try your best to cope. Enjoy seeing new sights that you can easily reach. These things will enhance the good memories you take home. Enjoy being away from home! Enjoy coming back home! When you are doing well, appreciate kind comments from others! Remember that when you receive genuine encouragement, it will help motivate your recovery.

8

Eight: Flying To a Resort after a Stroke

As I have mentioned, after I could drive again, my confidence level increased so much that I was ready to make arrangements to fly to a warm Caribbean island between Thanksgiving and Christmas, when the travel rates are low. I did not have any medical reasons not to travel, but I had apprehensions and fears. Still, I made the arrangements myself, using a travel agent who has successfully flown us many places. We made reservations to stay at a resort for ten days.

I was thrilled that I had travel plans. Travel adds so much to my life. I enjoy watching people in new surroundings. I enjoy hearing different opinions about issues. I enjoy doing different physical things. Before I had a stroke, Ken and I traveled extensively. Sometimes I traveled alone, usually to professional meetings. Whenever we came home, we brought different perspectives to our lives. That made our experience base "richer," because we appreciated different cultures.

When I taught my undergraduate class, "World Food and You," I always encouraged my students to travel. Many came back years later and told me about interesting places in the world they had visited. Traveling was a very rewarding aspect of my academic career. When I lectured, I included as much as I could about what I had eaten in other parts of the world. My father was in the Norwegian Merchant Marine, and had sailed to many seaports throughout the world. During lectures, I told my students about advice my father had given me, "If you are given meat, and you do not know what it is, do not ask!" I continually gave my students lectures about food safety around the world.

As we import so many foods to the U.S., many

other countries are required to follow our food laws if they want to sell foods to us. One of my graduate students is employed by the Food and Drug Administration (FDA), where his primary role is to inspect imported foods. In addition to being safe, they must be grown with herbicides and antibiotics approved in the United States. In Mexico, I have been in processing plants where the areas are partitioned and the area for the U.S. is separated from other areas. If you purchase an orange from South Africa, know that the FDA has screened these foods using random inspections. With each day, the quantity of imported foods increases. As a society, we like having a wide variety of foods to select from.

When my students visited Mexico during Spring Break, I told them to brush their teeth in beer instead of water. They grinned, and maybe they paid attention. I cautioned my students to think about their personal safety first, but explore rich and poor areas of the countries they visit. I also gave them advice about who "ugly Americans" are. That term is used by other countries when they see people from the U.S. very uncomfortable in foreign countries. They want things like they are used to, and make ridiculous demands. I used to give an entire 50-minute lecture about things I have observed "ugly Americans" do. I hope none of my previous students function in that capacity.

We Required Three Flights

I wondered about finding the right flight number and the time of departure and arrival. Although Ken was traveling with me, I did not want to be reliant on his advice alone. Our warm destination required three flights, two to get there and one to come home. Starting at 5 a.m. was no problem, as I slept on the initial flight. Walking through the airport after the first flight was difficult, as I had to go up and down escalators, keeping within the security area. I had avoided escalators since my stroke. I followed along behind Ken. I know elevators are always there for use, but we had to get to our second plane in a hurry. The down escalators were the worst.

We made it on the second plane and I enjoyed seeing the ocean below. I was looking forward to the warmth that was ahead. When we landed at our destination, I was hoping the plane would have a skyway. But, there was none, and climbing down the stairs from a 757 plane is a long way down. I slowly went down the stairs, hanging on tightly, remembering the advice from my physical therapist. As I got to the ground, there was a kind attendant looking very concerned. She took my hand and I said, "I made it."

The departing flight from our resort left at 11 p.m., and I was naturally exhausted, not looking forward to returning to snow and ice. Climbing up the stairs to the 757 was much easier than climbing down. One passenger was in a wheel chair. A forklift carried him up to the door of the plane. He was well strapped in. Other people travel with difficulties more serious than mine.

On that flight, I had a panic attack for about 30 minutes, which I had never had before. Ken said that my face looked strange and my right side shook. I gulped down a glass of 7-UP, but it did not help. I wanted to get out of that plane! Ken was afraid I might be having another stroke. So, I got Ken to talk to me for the next three hours and I responded okay. I knew that one sign of a stroke is that you cannot talk, so we had a silly conversation!

Finally, the plane landed and I could get off. I was fine. The next day I had my Coumadin level checked by my physician. It was within the normal range, so I would not have had a stroke on that flight. I requested a prescription for a tranquilizer I could carry with me on planes in case I ever have another anxiety attack.

Having Fun at the Resort

The island to which we traveled had left-side driving with loads of hills and winding roads. We decided to use taxis, instead of a rental car. We were driven to a beautiful resort at a great location on the island. We could swim on the sandy beach. We could sit under palm trees and eat or drink at the outdoor restaurant near the beach. We could snorkel, as there were rocks on both sides of the beach. The beach had a raft to which I could easily swim. I loved swimming in the ocean and feeling the salt on my skin.

Our suite was about seven levels from the beach. The walkways were not level, and the stair widths differed, so I used my left side with caution, making sure I hung onto the railings. Again, I always thought about advice from my physical therapist. Many of the railings were at different heights.

I agreed not to try snorkeling because I knew that adding a flipper to my left leg would probably exert it too much. Also, I wanted to swim close to shore. To me, there are few pleasures as great as swimming in salt water. On some days, we had good waves, and on other days the sea was very calm. I did not have any difficulty swimming. I cannot tell you whether or not I swam in a straight line, because I was not in a pool and it did not matter. I saw many swimmers who swam as well as I used to be able to.

The water temperature was 79° F. The sand was nice and warm. We could not have asked for more. Ken had a great time snorkeling and he did not have to be concerned about me. Previously, we had always snorkeled together. Ken came back with tales about a large turtle and different fish he had seen. I thought it was important that he had a break from worrying.

Ken always waited patiently for me to come up the considerable distance to our suite or when I came down to the beach below. Sitting on our balcony and watching the ocean gave me tremendous pleasure. Having grown up near the ocean, I am always thrilled when I see it again. Having what I had experienced since February 26, 2003, it was important for me to have some real fun and not be so concerned about myself. I needed to see different things and enjoyed meeting people.

Traveling To a Duty-Free Town

One day I went shopping while Ken went sightseeing. That is our usual procedure when we travel. I enjoy watching people and shopping and hearing later about Ken's adventures. We took a taxi to town and agreed on a time and location to meet after we split up. I went into stores to ask owners for their suggestions about where to eat. With left-hand driving, I crossed the streets with caution. I was able to understand their directions and found the correct restaurants. As usual, Ken used maps to get his directions. Men never want to ask for directions! Having a cell phone would have made this much easier, but that is for next time.

The Mile-Long Beach

Ken and I took a taxi to a beach which was defined as "the most beautiful beach in the world." I have seen plenty of beaches defined in this way, but this one we wanted to enjoy. We were walking along the beach from end-to-end, enjoying the pelicans and the high waves. I was feeling glad that I had exercised so much so that I could enjoy this beach, with the waves crashing in. Unfortunately, we stopped for some ice cream.

A Huge Iguana

A huge iguana was at the ice cream stand. He was about 3½ feet long and was the most horrible creature I have ever seen. As you know, I appreciate animals, but not this kind. Ken was watching the iguana climb up a tree as we walked back to the sand. Instead of watching where I was walking, I was watching the iguana. I did not see the roots of the tree. So, I fell and twisted my left ankle. I hobbled into the ocean to swim, but the pain was too much. We had to go back to our suite for ice! I was being so careful, but not careful enough. Luckily, I had packed a bandage and I had fallen on sand! Being on Coumadin gave me a terrible bruise. I was lucky I had not fallen on concrete. That was the first fall since my stroke.

Another Island

After falling, I took more time getting up and

down to our suite. As soon as I could walk without much difficulty, our plans were to take a ferry to another small island. The island had a park on it, so our initial plans were to hike in the park and swim or snorkel. As I could not hike, Ken went hiking and snorkeling. I debated about what I should do as we had heard the second island was gorgeous. I looked at the tourist information and found a taxi with twenty seats that went around the entire island. I decided that was what I would do. I did not want to be considered one of those "old" people who just drive around, but I had no other option. I thoroughly enjoyed the taxi ride around the island, and saw the place where Ken was snorkeling. Ken had a good time but I saw more of the island than he did. It was a highlight! I was given a thorough explanation of the entire island. Ken said the beach where he snorkeled was even better than the one we had gone to where I fell. At first I was disappointed that I had had an accident, but I was glad that I figured out how to have a pleasant time. Now when anyone asks me if I have seen that island, I can tell them that I have seen the entire thing, and direct them to things they want to see.

My insurance company gave me coverage for one year after my stroke, which is a wonderful benefit of many insurance plans because people do have accidents when they are not as strong as they used to be. About a month after my fall, I went to a physical therapist to get help with my ankle. It was still badly bruised. I had gone to her before. She asked, "Did you fall on the ice?" I had to tell her about the ugly iguana! My physical therapist prescribed the needed therapy to speed up my healing.

Returning Home Again

An interesting event happened when we returned home. The day after we returned, we were having a Christmas dinner for our Gourmet Club. Before we left, I had planned the table settings and had all the china ready. Our house cleaner was going to shampoo the carpets and have the house cleaned and ready for our party. All members of our group were going to bring the food. All Ken and I had to do was set the table. Everyone was amazed when they learned that we had returned home the day before. They were pleased to hear about our travels. They were jealous that they had not experienced a warm island. This gave me a subtle feeling that, "I could do anything." However, I must admit that I was tired!

Your Enlightenment

I am so glad that I went on vacation! Swimming, shopping and the scenery were wonderful. Anyone can have an accident! Being away from ice and snow was a delight! I now have prescribed medicine if I ever get another anxiety attack. My apprehensions did not occur. I feel free to travel again. I am glad that Ken was with me.

When you travel, be sure that you have a good travel agent who will make all the arrangements. If you need a wheelchair or have trouble walking, have an attendant meet you and take you to your next flight in the airport. Travel with a companion. Airports are difficult with the additional pressure of finding your next flight.

Go and see places you will enjoy. Be as physically careful possible. Do not go until you feel sure that you are ready to enjoy new places. When I sent some scenery pictures from the island to my uncle, his comment was, "You found peace and serenity!" This was an "easy" trip, as we only went to one location for ten days.

9

Nine: Stress and Success

Everything discussed in this book could cause extensive levels of stress, which is a very destructive force for your body to function well. I used to observe the effects of stress when my students took an examination. The more worried they were, the less well they did on exams. Some students were so stressed that they got drunk the night before the exam. Others would say that they did not think they would do well, so they went to a movie the night before. Generally, the students who enjoyed the movie had better scores, as their level of stress was less.

Coping With Stress

I do not like to use the word "coping," but there is no better word.

Stress is something you must deal with after a stroke. You have to realize that the initial reactions of fear and devastation will disappear. You have to believe that all the activities you are taught will be remembered. You will do them slowly at first and have to believe that your speed will eventually increase. You have to concentrate. You have to be persistent. You have to pay attention to details.

One major cause of stress is that you do not know how long the effects of a stroke will last. Everyone will tell you that all strokes are different. I was furious when I was constantly told that! One thing that has helped me the most was writing this book to give advice. We live in the "Show-Me State" of Missouri. I guess I have adopted their motto by the actions I have taken to understand why I have stress and endeavor to decrease it. Recovery from a stroke is a long process. You get rewards from improvements in little steps.

Many Silly Examples of Stress

Reducing stress levels made me feel more competent. One solid piece of advice I can give is that pressure is one of the things that makes stress worse. I have included many silly examples in this chapter when I was dealing with stress. Some of you can probably do them easily without stress, but they stress me. None of these examples would have caused me stressed before I had a stroke.

Ironing a Suit

One day I had to wear a silk suit and look spiffy. I had an awful time ironing it. I gave a really rough verbal time to our cats, instead of Ken, who was fortunately outdoors. Next time the suit goes to the dry cleaners for pressing. Many people have told me that there is usually an alternative way of getting things done. Using a dry cleaners is definitely one of them.

Word-Processing this Manuscript

I had problems word-processing this manuscript

and Ken would have to come to help me. Occasionally, I just laughed at my mistakes. Sometimes I just felt foolish and frustrated. Frequently I found a cat to stroke. I have an office desk with two top drawers on either side. In the drawers, I have afghans that my mother knitted for me. Sorrento sits in the drawer on my left-hand side, and Tofino sits in the drawer on my right-hand side. Comox sits on a couch in front of my desk. The cats are trained to never go on my desk and therefore never touch my computer. I have heard that cats cannot be trained, but I do not believe that.

So, whenever I want, when I am trying to think about the right words to use, I stroke a cat and contemplate. For me, their purrs greatly relieve my stress. Finally, when I had completed the entire rough draft, and Ken looked at it, he realized that I was not completely capable of word-processing, as I had too many spelling and indenting mistakes. When I told my Norwegian friend over the telephone, she said, "Well, you silly thing, you have had a stroke!" So, the way I looked at it is that I would put all my organized thoughts down, and somebody else would do the "mechanics" of word processing. When I told my former secretary that I was going to write this book and word-process it myself, she laughed and laughed, because I had never learned how to word-process before I had a stroke. I always gave her rough drafts that she perfected.

At the Post Office

Going to the Post Office is always a frustrating experience. When you finally make it to the front of the long line, the postal employee asks so many questions! Do you want priority or airmail? Do you have your customs forms prepared? Do you need insurance? Do you need any other stamps?

And when you find your credit card, they want to know if it is debit or credit. People in the line behind you are waiting for your answers. I am pressured! I never tell anyone who does not know me I have had a stroke. I believe that fact should be kept private.

Being on Time

Reading the clock and easily judging time is still a challenge. Time is always a problem, so I have to leave home with ample time to get to an appointment. I frequently look at the clock and plan when to leave. My goal is to always be on time. I am very stressed when I think I am going to miss an appointment.

Elevators vs. Escalators

I try to use elevators because coming down an escalator scares me, as I am afraid of falling. Wherever there is an escalator, there is usually an elevator close to it. In clothing stores, I usually find other items on sale when I look for the elevator.

Driving Without Stress

I knew I could not be stressed when driving. So, at first I drove in good weather and took short familiar trips before I got too tired. I have never let driving stress me. I do not talk on a cell phone or use the radio when I am driving, and always allow ample time to reach my destination.

Using Libraries

Given the problem I have with numbers, I find libraries terribly frustrating. In public libraries, I usually find it easier to go to the reference desk for assistance. A colleague sent me a list of ten scientific references he wanted copies of, which were in our main library on campus. I went to the science librarian and told her that I had had a stroke and could not easily deal with numbers. I told her that I could find these references, but it would take hours. She knew me and was glad to help. She found the references and then helped copy and collate them because I was having difficulty counting the pages. She assured me that is part of the service that reference librarians are directed to do. I was glad I had not struggled alone. What I learned from this experience was that I could have done it alone, but getting help was really appreciated, and I knew my colleague got the articles that he required and they were properly collated.

Having Parties

At first, my stress level was such that I felt very uncomfortable in groups, and the stress level was intense for about eight months after my stroke. It has now disappeared. I just did not want to be in academic situations, where I would not be familiar with current issues, and make a fool of myself. When I am in unfamiliar surroundings, my level of stress is higher and I become frustrated!

The simplest things frustrate me, as I think so slowly!

Trouble with Zippers

The only zipper that I have been able to do without difficulty is the zipper on the dome over our swimming pool. When I dress in a hurry, I have to concentrate on that damned zipper. Zippers on luggage are nothing more than a frustration. I sometimes wonder if an occupational therapist had given me zipper training on the rehabilitation unit in the hospital if I would still have the same problem.

Long Things Like Hoses and Extension Cords

Two long things really bother me. First, what end of the hose do I connect to the faucet? Secondly, what end of the long extension cord should be plugged in? I know children are told about the male and female ends of an extension cord and they learn it forever. When I discussed this issue with a friend, she made the statement about children, and said I must be so frustrated. Being referred to as a child again really hurt!

These two situations are probably connected somewhere in my brain as I also had trouble figuring out which end of our 75-foot long pool I should go to be able to roll up the cover. I have trouble with everything that is long! One end functions, the other end does not. So, why do I have trouble figuring out which end to use? I cannot answer that simple question, and continue to make mistakes with all of those long things. I think reaching a level of success is going to take a long time before choosing the correct end. I just persist until I get it right. You can imagine how silly I must look! I am not looking forward to putting lights on our Christmas tree.

If I were to ask Ken to list everything that stressed me, this chapter would never end. This book could be filled with the funny things my slow memory makes me do.

Reducing Your Stress

Swimming is wonderful therapy. As I have said, when I was working, "I wrote lectures as I swam." Recently, I wrote this book for you. Having a feeling of success reduced my stress level. There are many techniques you can personally use to calm down. Determine what reduces your stress level. Activities that should not be considered include eating too much, excessive alcohol consumption, or illegal drugs.

Some people are taught self-hypnosis, which

helps them. Some people try yoga. After reading this book, I am sure you have realized that my sense of humor helped me cope with stress. Being persistent about everything eventually helped reduce my level of stress. **I tend to concentrate more on success rather than stress.**

My Continual Stress

One of the things that I find constantly annoying is telling a friend something ridiculous I have done and they say, "I have done that, too." I laugh and say something nice, but this is annoying because, before I had a stroke, I would not have made such an error. I believe that I will have to deal with this situation for the rest of my long life.

Your Enlightenment

Know that being persistent and successfully overcoming challenges will reduce your level of stress. Many different things are stressful. I hope you laugh at my examples. Do not let stress overcome you. You will have many opportunities ahead when you will not even think about the time you suffered a stroke. The feeling is wonderful when you tell people you have met for the first time that you had a stroke, and they find that hard to believe! Perhaps you could make a list of the silly things you did because of pressure and stress, and keep it for one month. Laugh at the list. The next month, you should write a much shorter list. Persistence in overcoming stress will lead to feelings of success.

10

Ten: Embracing My Retirement Life

When people ask me if I am enjoying my retirement, and I tell them that I had a stroke, some say, "And look what happened after you retired." They are implying that terrible things happen to persons who have just retired. All that I have told you about my stroke occurred after I retired. I want to continue to have the best quality of life that is possible. My professional retirement goal was to be on an international committee for the Institute of Food Technologists (IFT). I received a letter on the day of my stroke inviting my membership on this committee. I did not have to attend a meeting with this committee until July

2003. When I was able to understand it all, as I have told you, I discussed it with my physician. He said that I would probably make so much progress by July 2003 that I should agree to be on the committee. My speech pathologist also said that she had been trying to get me ready for the July meeting, but she personally wondered if she would be able to do it.

Receiving this letter made me feel very good. In May 2003, I started making travel arrangements for the July meeting. That was impossible for me to do, as I arranged to arrive a day after the committee had met. I wondered if I had made a good decision. Ken was thinking about my affirmative decision, but did not say anything to me. He knew how much I was looking forward to serving on this committee and he did not want to deter me if it were not necessary.

Then, an important event happened. IFT was undergoing strategic planning and my committee was disbanded before they even met. I was very relieved! I was given the opportunity to join another international committee with IFT, which had a very detailed list of activities. The area it would be working with included the Department of Homeland Security, the increasing volume of imported foods, changing quality and safety guidelines, labeling for nutriceuticals and diet supplements, genetically modified foods, USDA regulations, Mad Cow Disease, documenting organic foods, food trade embargoes, water issues, and international food regulations. All of these activities will have an impact on our global food supply. I decided that I could not effectively function on that committee.

By reading the functions listed above, I hope you notice how far-reaching the effects of food science are. I would have to be in charge of some subcommittees, read numerous scientific articles that would involve statistics, and give presentations at large meetings. I had to realize that I could not understand statistical presentations. I could probably not find the references in our university library. Many prestigious scientists were assigned to that committee. I regret that I did not get to know them. So, as a result of my stroke, my academic life ended. I had spent my academic life working in these areas, so I really struggled with my decision to decline. One of the most important realizations was that it was important to end my academic career before I was seen as out of touch because of my lack of up-to-date information. I have seen many professors not step back from their careers in time. If you know college students, I am sure you can remember them telling you that a professor was "over the hill." By my decision, nobody was going to say that I was not current, and fortunately, I was not going to give any wrong information that could have hindered the actions of this international committee. They have a large charge and I wish them loads of success meeting their challenges. **Still, it was a great honor to be invited**.

I was recognized as one of eighteen "Innovators for the Millennium in 2000" in *U.S. News and World Report* (Volume 128, Number 1) for my public health contributions. Although I had to end my academic career in 2003, I hoped the seventeen others recognized in that issue would enjoy long careers in the millennium. I just have to be satisfied with what I was able to accomplish before 2000, which enabled me to get that important recognition.

A Good Party at Home

Ken and I had our first retirement party on February 27, 2004. We told our friends that I had heart surgery on February 26, 2000, and a stroke on February 26, 2003. So, it was time to have a party! Few people remembered that both had occurred on the same calendar day. As I could not cope with a party on Canada Day – Independence Day, this would be our first party. We invited about 40 friends. Everybody likes doing something in February, so they all accepted. Ken started preparing for guests on Monday by putting gravel on our long driveway, as country living has its own challenges with mud.

We planned the menu, and Ken established a food production schedule. He said, "I am in charge." I did basic KP duties. By 1:30 p.m. on Friday afternoon, all the food was cooked and the table looked gorgeous. Our guests were not coming until 6:30 p.m. At previous parties, I did a large share of the work. This time, Ken made everything from scratch and everyone was amazed at the food that was displayed. I enjoyed saying that Ken had prepared everything.

I received many comments like, "I have never seen you look better" and "You really look lovely tonight." Obviously, these comments made me feel good. Nobody could observe that my left side did not feel perfectly normal. As I had not been walking too much, I did not have a limp. Nobody asked me any logistical questions that I could not handle. We had a lot of fun that evening. One of the celebration cards that I received had the comment: "Your recoveries are due to the strengths within you working hard each day." That was a sincere comment that I will remember. A thank you note said: "What a great party! And what a great reason for celebration. Nan, you have gone through a lot these past few years and you have made it. You two make a great team."

Cooking with an Order

When I worked, I would wonder what I was going to cook for dinner as I drove home. I always prepared something for Ken, but I did not plan anything ahead. By January 2004, I was using the same approach. I was forgetting to cook part of our meals, like green beans to have with meat. So Ken insisted that we adopt a "retirement approach" and be organized. We began to thoroughly plan our meals.

When I am in the kitchen, I need help with complicated recipes. I can prepare everything, but I have to read the recipe and carefully follow all the directions. We often cook together. I mention this, because I had a habit of not thinking about dinner until I came home. I can no longer use this method. My stroke has forced me to learn to be prepared, or dinner can be a disaster.

My Enlightenment

I changed this "take-away" to *My Enlightenment* instead of *Your Enlightenment* because I want to stress my personal goals. Your goals will be much different, so I suggest you write your own section called *Your Enlightenment*. I will continue to keep myself healthy and fit. I will swim for 20 minutes every day with Ken as my lifeguard. I will keep my personal goal of not being too dependent on Ken. I will continue to struggle with math until I realize that further exercises will not help. I will continue to read articles in *Foreign Affairs* and other books and articles of interest. As I have mentioned earlier, I intend to learn how to do crossword puzzles. I will have fun with my friends and family, participate in a service organization, and travel as much as possible. In doing so, I hope I stimulate others to recover from stroke as much as it is possible. I will continue to stroke our cats! When this book is published, I will give copies to my friends and family, and I will sign it and write, "Do everything you can do to prevent having a stroke."

Epilogue

I did not include how my faith has sustained me when I wrote this book. I often thought that God got me out of the swimming pool so I could help others. Perhaps by writing this book, I am doing so. That is my hope. I am a confirmed Anglican and attend church and church-related service activities.

One other service I want to mention is that I was the President of the Scandinavian Heritage Society in Columbia, Missouri for nine years, many of those years after my stroke.

It became apparent when people asked me questions, that I had lost my food science memory.

No other parts of my memory were affected. I told a biologist friend about my loss and I used the example that I could not give the pH of a tomato. She asked me if it was acidic or basic, and I stumbled with my answer. I used to study *E coli*. Now all I can remember is that hamburgers have to be cooked until they are well done. Food science was the last thing I learned in college. I heard of a veterinary student who, after defending his Ph.D., had a stroke and lost his veterinary memory. He had to retake all his courses so that he could become a vet. The brain is certainly a complex organ.

I have had two accidents since the iguana incident on our island vacation. In Kansas City, I fell down four wood stairs (in the dark) and fractured the first cervical bone in my neck. I had to wear a neck brace during the six months of healing. When I was still in the Emergency Room, I asked a physician if I could still go to Italy in two weeks. His reply was, "Yes, but tell the pilot not to put the brakes on too hard."

When I travel in Europe, I use a hiking staff that fits in my suitcase, because I am afraid of the uneven cobblestones and my lack of balance. One day when Ken and I were enthralled with Pompeii, I had my neck brace on and was using my hiking staff. Suddenly, someone in the crowd shouted out, "You made it!" I do not know who she was, but it was a very kind thing for her to say. I guess she was associated with rehabilitation. I will always remember her statement. When my neck brace was removed, I went to physical therapy to help strengthen my neck.

The second accident occurred when I was sleepwalking. I fell in our bedroom at 4:30 a.m. that resulted in a compressed fracture of my 12th lumbar vertebra. Ken called 911 and two fire trucks and an ambulance came within five minutes. The staff inn the Emergency Room at Boone Hospital Center took x-rays and an MRI. An orthopedic surgeon told me that he could fix it with hot glue. I asked him if he had done this before, and he assured me that he had done it thousands of times. They made a small hole in my back near my 12th lumbar, and hot glue was injected. As it was so hot, all of the pain in my nerves also disappeared. Practicing good body mechanics when sitting up, I was able to go home at 3 p.m. without any pain. I started physical therapy again to learn how to strengthen my back. Within two weeks after my fall, I was on a whale watching excursion in a rolling boat off the coast of Newfoundland. I had been informed that the hot glue procedure was only effective with my type of injury if treatment was sought immediately. I felt very fortunate that I had gotten to the Emergency Room in time.

I requested physical therapy because I had learned about the benefits during rehabilitation. Under the care of the physical therapist, I started lifting 10 pounds the next day, but with a lot of pain. Today, I can easily lift 45 pounds, which I am slowly increasing on my own, at the Country Club of Missouri. My physical therapist told me to come back to see him once I got stronger. I liked the fact that he knew that I would continue to improve when he was not directly supervising me. Today, I alternate between swimming one day and lifting weights the next.

Last fall, I talked with a dear friend who I jogged with years ago. I told her that I spend half my life exercising. Her remark was simple "If you do not do that, you could not do any international traveling." She had a heart attack and died the next day, so that was the last thing she said to me.

I'll move on to brighter things. I am still an active member of the Fortnightly Club, Faculty Women and Wives of the University of Missouri-Columbia. I am in their Walking Group and we walk every Monday morning. We do not pay any attention to weather, we just walk. On narrow paths, I use my hiking staff. I have a chronic limp due to the fact that the nerve endings in my left foot were affected by my stroke. I have tried Anodyne Therapy (an infrared heat source), which only works to a limited extent, so walking with a limp is just part of my life. I am a member of the Fortnightly Club's Gourmet Study Group. I have no problem planning menus, but when Ken and I have to bring a dessert to a dinner, it is Ken's delight to prepare it. I am also a member of their Book Review Group, and have actually reviewed some books to an informal audience. The first one I did was a disaster, but I have gotten better since. I often wonder what the members would think if they could have seen me read my first *Wall Street Journal* article after my stroke. Now, perhaps they will read about it.

Ken and I enjoy attending many concerts and plays. We are fortunate to live in a university town with diverse cultural activities. We are frequently dinner guests of friends in their homes.

We built a home designed for entertaining, so we often have dinner parties at home. Ken is always "in charge", so everything gets done in time. I come up with the idea, invite the guests, arrange the menu and take care of all KP duties. Ken is organized and coordinated, so everything gets prepared at the right time. When we are not entertaining, I slowly cook all of our meals and leave the breads and pastries to Ken.

Since my stroke, Ken and I have traveled in Europe, several Caribbean Islands, and Canada. I have traveled alone three times, and have not had any problems. I just followed the advice I gave in Chapters Seven and Eight. I had to ensure that my travel agent made all of the arrangements. I enjoy the feeling of traveling alone, as I did when going to professional meetings.

Ending this Epilogue, I have to say Ken had to learn to live with a different person, as I think so slowly, which is personally frustrating. When I meet people for the first time, I am rewarded when they tell me that they had no indication that I had a stroke. **Thousands of people have much more difficulty than I do. I have great empathy for them.**

Appendix

Helpful Contacts: Here is a list of organizations that may be helpful. If you locate them on Google, you will learn that many of them have offices in your town or city. They will supply you with self-help literature. Often a visit to one of their offices will let you meet committed people who will assist you. Your local hospital will also be a good source for advice.

CANADA

(RESOURCES)

Canadian Association of Occupational Therapists

www.caot.ca

Canadian Association of Speech-Language Pathologists and Audiologists

www.caslpa.ca

Canadian Physiotherapy Association

www.physiotherapy.ca / www.thesehands.ca

Heart and Stroke Foundation of Canada

www.heartandstroke.com

Improving Stroke Recovery

www.abilitycamp.com/stroke.html

Speech Therapy for Stroke

www.communicationpartner.com

Stroke Caregivers

www.hope4stroke.com

Therapeutic Recreation Associations and Organizations

www.recreationtherapy.com/trorg.htm

USA

(RESOURCES)

American Academy of Neurology

www.aan.com

American Academy of Physical Medicine and Rehabilitation

www.aapmr.org

American Congress of Rehabilitation

www.acrm.org

American Occupational Therapy Association

www.aota.org

American Speech-Language-Hearing Association

www.asha.org

The American Therapeutic Recreation Association

www.atra-online.com

Family Caregiver Alliance

www.caregiver.org

National Institute of Neurological Disorders and Stroke

www.ninds.nih.gov

National Alliance For Caregiving

www.caregiving.org

USA

(RESOURCES CONTINUED)

National Stroke Association

www.stroke.org

National Organization for Empowering Caregivers

www.care-givers.com

National Family Caregivers Association

www.nfcacares.org

Visiting Nurses Service

www.vnsny.org /living with stroke

According to the American Heart Association, the signs of a stroke include:

1. Sudden numbness or weakness in the face, arm, or leg, especially on one side of the body.
2. Sudden confusion, trouble speaking or understanding.
3. Sudden trouble seeing in one or both eyes.
4. Sudden trouble walking, dizziness, loss of balance or coordination.
5. Sudden, severe headache.

If you think someone is having a stroke, here are the actions to follow immediately:

1. Ask the person to smile.
2. Ask the person to speak a simple sentence.
3. Ask the person to raise both arms.
4. Ask the person to stick out their tongue, If it is crooked and goes from one side to the other that is an indication of a stroke.

If this person fails at these, immediately take him or her to an Emergency Room or call 911. At times, if medication can be given soon, the effects of enduring what I had will be avoided.

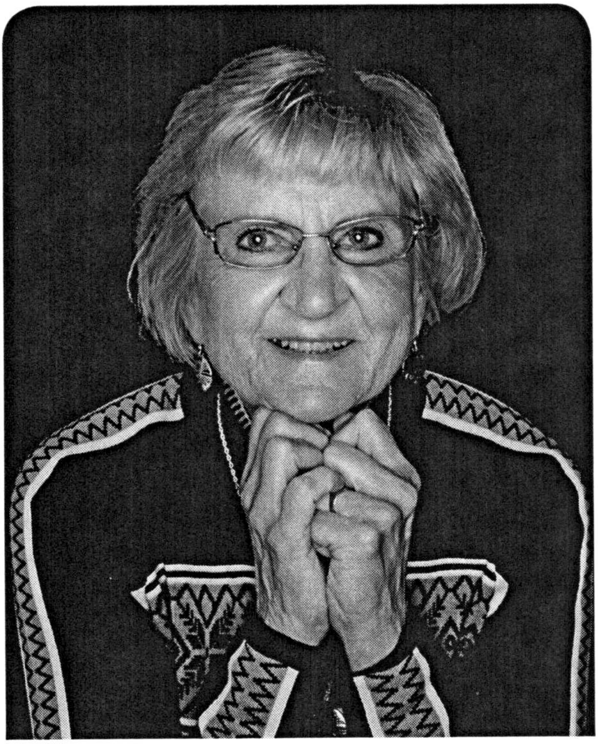

About the Author

Nan Unklesbay is a Professor Emeritus in Food Science at the University of Missouri-Columbia. She was featured as one of eighteen "Innovators For The Millennium" for her research in public health by *U.S. News & World Report* January 3 - 10, 2000. She suffered a profound stroke in 2003. Her strong recovery has lead to a different and very fulfilling life. She lives with her husband in Columbia, Missouri.

CPSIA information can be obtained at www.ICGtesting.com
Printed in the USA
LVOW10s1612130314

377300LV00007B/673/P

9 780984 228874